KETO RECIPES AND MEAL
PLANS FOR BEGINNERS

KETO FOR
LIFE

*Beautiful Ketogenic Diet
Recipes That Deliver A Punch
As Well As Weight Loss*

LORENA MUELLER

The information in the following pages is broadly considered to be a truthful and accurate account of facts and as such any inattention, use or misuse of the information in question by the reader will render any resulting actions solely under their purview. There are no scenarios in which the publisher or the original author of this work can be in any fashion deemed liable for any hardship or damages that may befall them after undertaking information described herein.

Additionally, the information in the following pages is intended only for informational purposes and should thus be thought of as universal. As befitting its nature, it is presented without assurance regarding its prolonged validity or interim quality. Trademarks that are mentioned are done without written consent and can in no way be considered an endorsement from the trademark holder.

Table of Contents

PART I

Chapter 1: The Keto Plan & How it Works

You will soon understand how you can eat most of the foods you always enjoy. You will be able to make some substitutes to get going which are described within this chapter.

Happy Discovery!

Several Types of Keto Diet Plans

- *Plan 1*: You can choose from the standard ketogenic diet (SKD) which consists of high-fat, moderate protein, and is extremely low in carbs.

- *Plan 2*: The cyclical ketogenic diet or CKD is created with 5-keto days trailed by two high-carb days.

- *Plan 3*: The targeted keto diet, which is also called TKD, will provide you with a plan to add carbs to the diet during the times when you are working out.

- *Plan 4*: The high-protein ketogenic diet is very similar to the standard keto plan in all aspects except that it has more protein.

However, let's not get too far ahead of the plan. You need to focus on the first 30 days! The long process to explain each of these types would take another entire book!

Health Benefits from a Ketogenic Diet Plan

These are just a few of the ways you can benefit from remaining on the diet plan. It's hard to believe a diet plan can remedy so many health issues.

Acne: Your insulin levels are lowered by consuming less sugar and eating less processed foods. The acne will begin to clear up as you continue with the plan.

Alzheimer's disease: The symptoms and progression will be slowed.

Lowered Blood Pressure: While using the keto plan; you are experiencing reduced intake of carbs which will reduce your blood pressure levels. It is recommended to seek advice from your regular doctor to see if it is possible to reduce some of your medication while you are on the keto diet. You may also have some dizziness when you first begin the plan which is one of the first indications that the plan is working. The result is a lack of carbohydrates.

Cancer: Slow tumor growths and several other types of cancer have shown improvement with the keto plan.

Diabetes and Pre-diabetes: The main link to pre-diabetes is excess body fat which is removed which is proven by research that insulin sensitivity was improved by as much as 70%.

Epilepsy: Children's research studies have proven the diet works in the reduction of seizure activity.

Gum Disease: The sugar you consume influences the pH balance in your mouth. If you have issues before you begin the plan; you should begin to see a remarkable improvement within approximately three months.

Obesity: When the ketogenic diet plan is followed—the weight will dissolve.

Stiffness and Joint Pain: It is important to continue with the elimination of any grain-based foods. It is believed that the grains are one of the largest factors which cause the pain. Just remember "no grain—no pain."

Thinking is Improved: You might be a bit foggy-minded when you first begin the plan since you will be consuming high-fat foods. After all, your brain is about 60% fat by weight; your thinking skills should improve with the intake of the fatty foods indicated with the keto diet.

The Elements of Ketosis

Ketosis is used to help your burn body fat and drop extra pounds. Proteins will fuel your body to burn the fat—therefore—the ketosis will maintain your muscles and make you less hungry.

Your body will remain healthy and work as it should. If you don't consume enough carbs from your food; your cells will begin to burn fat for the necessary energy instead. Your body will switch over to ketosis for its energy source as your cut back on your calories and carbs.

Two elements that occur when your body doesn't need the glucose:

Lipogenesis: If there is a sufficient supply of glycogen in your liver and muscles, any excess is converted to fat and stored.

Glycogenesis: The excess of glucose converts to glycogen and is stored in the muscles and liver. Research indicates that only about half of your energy used daily can be stored as glycogen.

As a result, your body will have no more food—similar to when you are sleeping—your body burns the fat and creates ketones. These ketones break down the fats, which generate fatty acids, and burn-off in the liver through beta-oxidation.

Simply stated, when you no longer have a supply of glycogen or glucose, ketosis begins and will use the consumed/stored fat as energy.

The Internet provides you with a keto calculator to use at http://keto-calculator.ankerl.com/. You can check your levels when you want to know what essentials your body needs during your diet plan or after. All you need to do is document your personal information such as weight and height. The calculator will provide you with the essential math.

Weight Loss and Protein

Protein needs to be in your plan for these reasons:

Protein is a Fat Burner: Science has proven your body cannot use and burn your fat as energy sources unless you have help from either carbs or protein. The balance of protein must be maintained to preserve your calorie-burning lean muscles.

Protein Saves Your Calories: Protein slows down your digestion process making you feel more satisfied from the foods you eat. During the first cycle of your diet plan; it is imperative that you feel full, so there is no temptation to cheat on the strategy.

Muscle Repair and Growth: Protein should be increased on days when you are more active. It is essential to have a plan on what your meals will consist of with

12

a balance of carbs, proteins, and calories. The balance is what you are attempting to achieve with a focused plan such as the keto diet.

The Role of Calories, Protein, and Carbs

Calories are held within your body with the use of the nutrients of protein, fat, and carbs which your body will use for energy.

Carbohydrates

Your body exchanges one-hundred percent of the carbs into glucose which gives your body an energy boost. About 50% to 60% of your intake of calories is produced by carbs. Carbs stored in your liver as glycogen is released as your body needs it. Glucose is essential for the creation of adenosine triphosphate (ATP) which is an energy molecule. The fuel from glucose is vital for the daily maintenance and activities inside your body. After the liver has reached its maximum capacity for its limits, the excessive carbohydrates turn into fat.

Count Those Carbs

Before you are totally in gear, you need to start carb counting to make sure you keep your body in perfect 'sync' with the plan. Reading the labels may be a bit nerve-racking in the beginning, but after a while, it will be as you have always done it that way.

Remember this Formula: Total Carbs minus (-) Fiber = Net Carbs

A rough estimate will include you consuming between 20 to 30 carbs daily. It is almost a necessity to own a set of food scales to take out the guesswork.

Keep this information in mind before you make the purchase:

- *The Automatic Shut-Off*: Seek a scale that does not have this option. The result could be you being in the midst of a recipe—move the dish—and the scale could reset; NOT.

- *The Tare Function*: When you set a bowl on the scale, the feature will allow you to reset the scale back to zero (0).

- *Removable Plate*: Keep the germs off of the scale by removing the plate. Be sure it will come off to eliminate the bacterial buildup.

- *Seek a Conversion Button*: You need to know how to convert measurements into grams since not all recipes have them listed. The grams keep the system in complete harmony.

Natural Supplements for Ketogenic Dieters

Fermented Foods: Use items, while on the keto plan such as coconut milk kefir, coconut milk, yogurt, pickles, sauerkraut, and kimchi to help with any digestive issues.

Lemon and Lime: Your blood sugar levels will naturally drop with these citric additions, and signal a boost in your liver function. Use them in green juices, with a salad, or with cooked with meats or veggies. The choices are limitless and assist you with the following:

- Reduces toothache pain

- Boosts your immune system

- Relieves respiratory infections

- Balances pH

- Decreases wrinkles and blemishes

- Reduces fever

- Excellent for weight loss

- Flushes out the unwanted, unhealthy materials

- Blood purifier

Apple Cider Vinegar: Who would believe the benefits you can receive from just one to two tablespoons of vinegar in an 8-ounce glass of water would help the process? You can choose the straight up method and skip the water. These are just a few ways this helps your progress:

- Reduces cholesterol

- Excellent for detoxification

- Helps you to drop the pounds

- Improves your digestion tract

- Helps with sore muscles

- Controls sugar intake/aids in diabetes

- Strengthens your immune system

- A good energy booster

- Balances your inner body system and functions

Cinnamon: Use cinnamon as part of your daily plan to improve your insulin receptor activity. Just put one-half of a teaspoon of cinnamon into a shake or any type of keto dessert. Many of the keto recipes contain the ingredient.

Turmeric: Dating back to Ayurveda and Chinese medicine the is of this Asian orange herb has been known for its anti-inflammatory compounds. Add it to you smoothies, green drinks, meats, or veggies. These are some of its benefits:

- Prevents Alzheimer's disease
- Weight management
- Relieves arthritis
- Reduces your cholesterol levels
- Helps control diabetes
- Improves your digestion

Be Aware of Some Foods and Beverages: Which Ones to Avoid

Agave Nectar: One teaspoon has 5 grams of carbs versus 4 grams in table sugar.

Beans and Legumes: This group to avoid includes peas, lentils, kidney beans, and chickpeas. If you use them, be sure to count the carbs, protein, and fat content.

Cashews and Pistachios: The high carb content should be monitored for these yummy nuts.

Fruits: Raspberries, blueberries, and cranberries contain high sugar contents. In small portions; you can enjoy some strawberries.

Grains and Starches: Avoid wheat-based items such as cereal, rice, or pasta.

Hydrogenated Fats: Cold-pressed items should be avoided when using vegetable oils such as safflower, olive, soybean, or flax. Coronary heart disease has been linked to these fats which also include margarine.

Tomato-based Products: Read the labels because most of the tomato products contain sugar. If you use them be sure to account for the sugar content. (The recipes provided have considered this.)

Chapter 2: The 14-Day Plan

Day One

Breakfast: Keto Scrambled Eggs

Ingredients

3 large eggs

Fresh ground pepper

Coarse salt

1 tablespoon unsalted butter

Instructions

1. Whisk the eggs in a bowl.

2. Use low heat and place the butter into a skillet.

3. Add the eggs. Continue to stir until well-done, usually 1 ½ to 3 minutes.

Serving Portion: Fat: 26.3 g; Carbs 1.8 g; Protein: 17.4 g; Calories: 318

Lunch: Tuna Cheese Melt (Low-Carbs)

Ingredients

2 Pieces of "Oopsie" bread

Ingredients for the Salad

1 to 2 Celery stalks

5 1/3 Tablespoons sour cream or mayonnaise

1 Can tuna (in olive oil)

4 Tablespoons chopped dill pickles

½ teaspoon lemon juice

Pepper and salt to taste

½ minced clove garlic

Toppings

A pinch of paprika powder or cayenne pepper

3 ½ ounces shredded cheese

Serving Ingredients

Olive oil

1/3 Pound leafy greens

"Oopsie" Bread (makes six to 8)

3 Eggs

A pinch of salt

4 ¼ ounces cream cheese

½ teaspoon baking powder

½ Tablespoon ground psyllium husk powder

Instructions

1. Preheat the oven to 350°F. Put parchment paper onto a cookie sheet.

2. Blend all of the salad ingredients.

3. Place the bread slices on the prepared sheet, spread the tuna, and sprinkle the cheese on top of each slice of bread.

4. Sprinkle some cayenne or paprika powder on the sandwich halves and bake in the oven for about 15 minutes.

5. Have some leafy greens with a drizzle of olive oil.

"Oopsie" Bread Instructions

1. Heat the oven to oven at 300°F.

2. Begin by separating the egg whites (whites in one bowl and yolks in the other).

3. Whisk the egg whites with the salt until peaks are formed.

4. Combine the cream cheese and egg yolks—add the baking powder and psyllium seed husk (making it more Oopsie type bread).

5. Blend/fold in the whites into the yolk mixture—keeping out the air in the whites of the eggs.

6. Place six or eight 'oopsies' on the paper-lined sheet.

7. Bake in the center oven rack, usually for 25 minutes or until browned.

Dinner: Chicken Smothered in Creamy Onion Sauce

Ingredients

1 whole green/spring onion

2 tablespoons or 1-ounce butter

4 chicken breast halves (skinless—boneless)

8 ounces sour cream

½ teaspoon sea salt

Note: The chicken should weigh approximately six ounces or 170 g for this recipe.

Instructions

1. In a large pan, melt the butter on the stovetop using the med-high setting. Lower the heat setting to med-low—put the chicken with the butter—cover and cook about ten more minutes.

2. Chop the onion using just the white and green sections.

3. Flip the breasts—cover and simmer—another 8 or 9 minutes (or until completely done).

4. Combine the onion, and continue cooking the chicken for another one or two minutes.

5. Take it off of the burner, and blend in the salt and sour cream.

6. Let the meal rest and flavors blend for five minutes.

Stir well and serve.

Day Two

Breakfast: Mock Mc Griddle Casserole

Ingredients

1 pound breakfast sausage

¼ cup flaxseed meal

1 cup almond flour

10 large eggs

6 tablespoons maple syrup

4 ounces cheese

4 tablespoons butter

¼ teaspoon sage

½ teaspoon each: onion & garlic powder

Instructions

1. Heat the oven to 350°F. Use parchment paper to line a 9 x 9-inch casserole dish.

2. Using medium heat; start cooking the breakfast sausage on the stove in a skillet.

3. Blend all of the dry (the cheese included) ingredients and add the wet ones.

4. Add four tablespoons of the syrup and blend well.

5. After the sausage is crispy brown—blend all of the ingredients; (the fat too).

6. Pour the mixture into the dish and sprinkle the remainder of the syrup on the top.

7. Bake for 45 to 55 minutes. Remove it and let it cool.

Yields: Eight Servings

Time Saving Tip: The casserole should be easy to remove by using the edge of the parchment paper.

Lunch: Brussels Sprouts with Hamburger Gratin

Ingredients

1 Pound Ground beef

1 Pound Brussels sprouts

½ Pound diced bacon

4 tablespoons sour cream

1/3 Pound shredded cheese

1- ¾ Ounces butter

Pepper and salt to taste

1 tablespoon Italian seasoning

Instructions

1. Cut the Brussels sprouts in half.

2. Preheat the oven to 425°F/220°C.

3. Saute the Brussels sprouts and bacon in the butter. Flavor with the sour cream and place in a baking pan/dish.

4. Fry the beef and season with pepper and salt; add the herbs and cheese—sprinkling on top of the base layer.

5. Bake on the center rack of the oven for fifteen minutes.

Serve with a dollop of mayonnaise and a fresh salad.

Yields: Four Servings

Dinner: Squash and Sausage Casserole

Ingredients

1 pound browned sausage

2 large eggs

1 medium zucchini (sliced & cooked)

2 medium summer squash (sliced & cooked)

1 teaspoon salt

½ teaspoon onion powder or ¼ cup dried minced onion

1 cup mayonnaise

1 package sugar substitute (or stevia)

¼ teaspoon pepper

1 ½ cups shredded cheddar cheese (divided)

¼ melted butter

Instructions

1. Pre-set the oven to 350°F.

2. Blend each of the ingredients except for one-half of a cup of shredded cheese.

3. Put the ingredients into a lightly greased oblong baking plate.

4. Sprinkle the remainder of cheese on the casserole.

5. Bake until lightly browned for approximately thirty minutes.

This casserole will easily serve 12 people with an amazing flavor you won't soon forget!

Day Three

Breakfast: Can't Beat it Porridge

Ingredients

1 cups almond or coconut milk

1 pinch salt

1 Tablespoon each:

- Sunflower seeds

- Chia Seeds

Instructions

1. Using a small saucepan on the stovetop, blend each of the components, and bring to a boiling. Lower the burner and cook slowly until the porridge is the consistency you desire

2. Garnish with some butter or milk. You can also add some fresh unsweetened berries or cinnamon.

Yields: One Serving

Time Saving Tip: Make it ahead of time using a big glass jar. Fill the jar with the following ingredients and shake them up. Each serving will correspond with three tablespoons for each serving.

These are the ingredients needed for the batch:

1 Tbsp. cinnamon

½ tsp. salt

1 1/4 cup each:

- Sunflower seeds

- Flaxseeds

- Chia seeds

Lunch: Salad From a Jar

Ingredients

1 (4-ounce) rotisserie chicken/smoked salmon/other protein

1 ounce each:

- Cucumber

- Cherry tomatoes

- Leafy greens

- Bell pepper

4 tablespoons olive oil or mayonnaise

½ Scallion

Instructions

1. Chop or shred the veggies and place the leafy greens to the bottom for a crunch followed by the colorful veggies. (You can also use some cauliflower or broccoli for a change of pace.)

2. Top it off with some of the grilled protein of your choice. You can also use cold cuts, tuna fish, mackerel or boiled eggs.

3. Cheese cubes, seeds, nuts, and olives are also healthy and colorful additions.

4. Add a generous amount of mayonnaise or salad dressing and enjoy!

Yields: One Serving

Dinner: Ham and Cheese Stromboli

Ingredients

1 large egg

1 ¼ cups shredded mozzarella cheese

3 tablespoons coconut flour

4 tablespoons almond flour

4 ounces of ham

1 teaspoon Italian seasoning

3 ½ ounces cheddar cheese

Instructions

1. Preheat the oven to 400°F.

2. Melt the mozzarella cheese in the microwave for one minute/alternating at ten-second intervals; stirring until melted.

3. In a mixing bowl, blend the coconut and almond flour with the seasonings.

4. Toss in the mozzarella on the top and work it in.

5. After the cheese has cooled; beat the egg and combine everything

6. On a flat surface; put some parchment paper, and add the mixture.

7. Use a rolling pin or your hands to flatten the mix.

8. Place several diagonal lines using a knife or pizza cutter. (Leave a row of approximately four inches wide in the center.

9. Alternate the layers using the cheddar and ham on the uncut space of dough until you have used all of the filling.

10. Bake for 15 to 20minutes or it is browned.

Day Four

Breakfast: Frittata with Cheese and Tomatoes

Ingredients

6 eggs

2/3 cup soft cheese (ex. Feta 3 ½ ounces or 100 g)

½ medium white onion (1.9 ounces or 55 g)

2/3 cup halved cherry tomatoes

2 tablespoons chopped herbs (ex. basil or chives)

1 tablespoon ghee/butter

Instructions

1. Heat the oven broiler to 400°F.

2. Place the onions on a greased, hot iron skillet, and cook with ghee/butter until slightly brown.

3. In a separate container, crack the eggs and add the salt, pepper, or add herbs of your choice. Whisk and add to the onion pan.

4. Cook until the edges begin to get brown. Top with the cheese and tomatoes.

5. Put the pan in the broiler for five to seven minutes or until done.

Lunch: Chicken—Broccoli—Zucchini Boats

For a variety textures as well as flavors to spice up lunch; this is the one!

Ingredients

6 ounces shredded chicken

2 tablespoons butter

2 hollowed-out zucchini (10 ounces)

3 ounces shredded cheddar cheese

1 stalk of green onion

1 cup broccoli

2 tablespoons sour cream

Instructions

1. Heat the oven temperature to 400°F.

2. Slice the zucchini lengthwise and scoop most of the insides out until you have a shell of approximately ½ to 1 cm. thick.

3. Melt one tablespoon of the butter into each boat, flavor with a dash of pepper and salt, and bake them for around twenty minutes.

4. Shred the chicken, cut the broccoli florets into small pieces, and measure out six ounces of cheese. Blend in with the sour cream.

5. Remove the zucchini shells when done and add the mixture.

6. Sprinkle each of them with the remainder of the cheese.

7. Bake for another ten or fifteen minutes until the cheese is browned and melted.

8. Use a bit of sour cream, mayonnaise, or chopped onion as a garnish.

Dinner: Steak-Lovers Slow-Cooked Chili

Ingredients for Chili:

1 cup beef or chicken stock

½ cup sliced leeks

2 ½ pounds (1-inch cubes) steak

2 cups whole tomatoes (canned with juices)

1 tablespoon chili powder

½ tsp. salt

1/8 tsp. ground black pepper

¼ tsp. ground cayenne pepper

½ tsp. cumin

Optional Toppings

1 teaspoon fresh chopped cilantro

2 tablespoons sour cream

¼ cup shredded cheddar cheese

½ avocado (cubed or sliced)

Instructions

1. Place all of the items except the topping fixings into the slow cooker.

2. Set the cooker on the high setting for about six hours.

Yields: Twelve Servings

Serving Portion: 1: Fat: 26.0 g; Carbs 3.3 g; Protein: 38.4 g; Calories: 321

Servings with Toppings. Serving Portion: 1: Fat: 41.32 g; Carbs 13.49 g; Protein: 32.47 g; Calories: 540.33

Day 5

Breakfast: Brownie Muffins

Ingredients

½ tsp. salt

1 cup flaxseed meal

¼ cup cocoa powder

½ Tbsp. baking powder

1 Tbsp. cinnamon

2 Tbsp. coconut oil

1 large egg

1 tsp. vanilla extract

¼ cup sugar-free caramel syrup

½ cup pumpkin puree

¼ cup slivered almonds

1 tsp. apple cider vinegar

Instructions

1. Heat the oven temperature at 350°F.

2. In a deep mixing bowl—combine all of the ingredients—mixing well.

3. Use six paper liners in the muffin tin, and add ¼ cup of the batter to each one.

4. Sprinkle several almonds on the tops, pressing gently.

5. Bake approximately fifteen minutes. It is done when the top is set.

Serving Portion: 1 muffin (The recipe serves six): Fat: 13.4 g; Carbs 8.2 g; Protein:

7 g; Calories: 183.3

Lunch: Bacon-Avocado-Goat Cheese Salad

Ingredients

½ Pound bacon

½ Pound goat cheese

4 ounces walnuts

2 avocados

4 ounces arugula lettuce

Ingredients for the Dressing

7 ½ tablespoons mayonnaise

Juice of ½ of a lemon

2 tablespoons heavy whipping cream

7 ½ tablespoons olive oil

Instructions

1. Preheat the oven temperature to 400°F/200°C.

2. Prepare a baking dish with some parchment paper.

3. Slice the goat cheese into ½-inch round slices and put in the baking dish. Place on the upper rack of the oven.

4. Pan-fry the bacon until crunchy.

5. Cut the avocados and place on top of a bed of lettuce, add the bacon, cheese, and nuts to the top of your creation.

6. Make the dressing using a stick blender. Sprinkle in a dash of pepper, salt, or a few fresh herbs.

Yields: Four Servings

Dinner: Tenderloin Stuffed Keto Style

Ingredients

2 pounds pork tenderloin or venison

½ cup feta cheese

½ cup gorgonzola cheese

1 teaspoon chopped onion

2 tablespoons crushed almonds

2 garlic cloves, minced

½ teaspoon each: fresh ground black pepper and sea salt

Instructions

1. Preheat the grill.

2. Form a pocket in the tenderloin.

3. Mix the cheeses, almonds, garlic, and onions.

4. Stuff the pocket, and seal using a skewer.

5. Grill until its desired doneness.

Yields: Eight Servings

Serving Portion: 1: Fat: 6.2 g; Carbs 2.9 g; Protein: 28.8 g; Calories: 194

Day 6

Breakfast: Sausage—Feta—Spinach Omelet

Ingredients

½ tablespoon extra-virgin olive oil

2 sausage links

3 large eggs

¼ cup Half & Half

1 cup spinach

1 tablespoon feta cheese

Note: You will need two skillets for this yummy omelet!

Instructions

1. Use medium heat for both pans, and pour olive oil in one of the two.

2. In a small dish, use the Half & Half and mix with the eggs—add the seasonings—and scramble.

3. In the clean pan, cook the sausage.

4. Sauté the spinach in the oiled pan—add a pinch of salt and pepper if desired.

5. After both have finished cooking; put them together in a bowl.

6. Transfer the olive oiled pan to the sausage fat pan—and add the eggs.

7. When the edges begin to cook—add the spinach, sausage, and cheese. Cook another minute—flip the omelet. Cook another two to three minutes.

8. Cover one pan with the other and let the combo steam.

9. Remove and enjoy your masterpiece!

Serving Portion: Fat: 43 g; Carbs 3 g; Protein: 31 g; Calories: 535

Lunch: Pancakes with Cream-Cheese Topping

Don't be alarmed, this is an excellent choice for any time and is so healthy.

Ingredients

8 ¾ ounces cottage cheese

5 eggs

1 tablespoon ground psyllium husk powder

A pinch of salt

For Frying: Coconut oil or butter

Ingredients for the Topping

2 tablespoons red or green pesto

½ pound (8 ounces) ricotta or cream cheese

2 tablespoons olive oil

Ground black pepper and Sea Salt

½ thinly sliced red onion

Instructions

1. Combine one tablespoon of the olive oil with the pesto and cream cheese; set aside.

2. Using a hand blender, mix the salt, cottage cheese, eggs, and husk powder; blend until smooth. Let rest for ten minutes.

3. On the stovetop using the medium heat setting; heat two tablespoons of the oil or butter.

4. Drop several dollops of the cheese batter (2 to 3 inches in diameter), frying the pancakes a few minutes per side.

5. Serve with a few red onion slices with a drizzle of oil, pepper, and salt. You can also use fresh herbs, smoked fish roe or chopped chives.

Dinner: Skillet Style Sausage and Cabbage Melt

Ingredients

4 spicy Italian chicken sausages

2 tablespoons coconut oil

½ cup diced onion

1 ½ cups purple cabbage

1 ½ cups green cabbage

2 tablespoons chopped fresh cilantro

2-1-ounce slices Colby jack cheese

Instructions

1. Start by removing the sausage casings and rough-chopping them. Shred the cabbage and chop the onions.

2. Add the coconut oil, cabbage, and onion in a large skillet using the med-high setting for approximately eight minutes (the veggies should be tender).

3. Blend the cheese and cover.

4. Turn the heat off and let it rest five minutes as the cheese melts.

5. When it is time to serve—stir gently and add the cilantro.

Yields: Four Servings

Serving Portion: 1: Fat: 14.62 g; Carbs 3.52 g; Protein: 18.26 g; Calories: 231

Day 7

Breakfast: Tapas

Have a great mixture!

Ingredients

Cold Cuts:

- Prosciutto
- Serrano ham
- Salami
- Chorizo

Cheeses:

- Gouda

- Parmesan

- Mozzarella

- Cheddar

Veggies:

- Pickled cucumbers

- Peppers

- Radishes

- Cucumbers

Avocado with pepper and homemade mayonnaise

Fresh Basil

Splash of fresh squeezed lemon juice

Nuts:

- Hazelnuts

- Almonds

- Walnuts

Instructions

1. Cut all of the ingredients into cubes or sticks and split the avocado cutting its fruit into small wedges.

2. Blend with four ounces of mayonnaise pepper and maybe a splash of lemon juice

3. Use the avocado shells for the serving platter.

Yields: Four Servings

Lunch: Tofu—Bok-Choy Salad

Tofu Ingredients:

15 ounces extra firm tofu

2 teaspoons minced garlic

Juice from ½ a lemon

1 tablespoon each:

- sesame oil

- water

- soy sauce

- rice wine vinegar

Bok Choy Salad Ingredients:

2 tablespoons soy sauce

1 stalk green onion

2 tablespoons chopped cilantro

9 ounces bok choy

3 tablespoons coconut oil

1 tablespoon Sambal Olek

Juice of ½ of a lime

1 tablespoon peanut butter

7 drops liquid Stevia

Instructions

1. Press the tofu in towels for approximately five to six hours to dry.

2. Combine each of the marinade ingredients.

3. When dry; chop the tofu into squares and put in a plastic container/bag with the marinade sauce.

4. Leave it to sit for at least thirty minutes—preferably overnight.

5. Heat the oven to 350°F. Bake for 30 to 35 minutes on a parchment paper-lined baking dish or a Silpat (non-stick baking sheet with a blend of fiberglass mesh and silicone).

6. In the interim, combine the dressing ingredients (except for the bok choy) in a mixing dish. Toss in the onion and cilantro.

7. Chop the bok choy as you would cabbage, into small slices.

8. Remove the tofu—combine, and enjoy.

Note: Bok choy is a Chinese vegetable.

Serving Portion: Fat: 35 g; Carbs 7.3 g; Protein: 25.0 g; Calories: 442.3

Dinner: Hamburger Stroganoff

Ingredients

8 ounces sliced mushrooms

1 pound ground beef

2 minced cloves of garlic

2 Tbsp. butter

1 ¼ cups sour cream

1/3 cup water or dry white wine

1 tsp. lemon juice

¼ tsp. paprika

1 tsp. dried parsley

Substitute: You may also use one tablespoon fresh chopped parsley.

Instructions

1. Sauté the onions and garlic in a skillet prepared using one tablespoon of butter.

2. Mix in the beef into the pan— sprinkle with pepper and salt if desired. Cook until done and set to the side.

3. Use the remainder of the butter, the mushrooms, and the wine/water, and add them to the pan. Cook until half of the liquid is reduced and the mushrooms are soft.

4. Take them off the burner—add the paprika and sour cream.

5. On low heat stir in the meat and lemon juice.

Use additional spices for flavoring if desired.

Serving Portion: 1 (272 g): Fat: 28.1 g; Carbs 6.1 g; Protein: 38.7 g; Calories: 447

Day 8

Breakfast: Cheddar—Jalapeno Waffles

Ingredients

3 large eggs

1 small jalapeno

3 ounces cream cheese

1 tablespoon coconut flour

1-ounce cheddar cheese

1 teaspoon each:

- baking powder

- Psyllium husk powder

Instructions

1. Combine all of the ingredients using an immersion blender (except for the jalapeno and cheese) until it has a smooth texture.

2. Add the cheese and jalapeno; blend and pour into the waffle iron.

3. You can garnish with your favorite ingredients in about five or six minutes total

Note: Psyllium husk is a native of Pakistan, Bangladesh, and India. It is available online at several locations

Serving Portion: 2 waffles: Fat: 28 g; Carbs 6 g; Protein: 16 g; Calories: 338

Lunch: Salmon Tandoori with Cucumber Sauce

Ingredients

1 ½ Pounds Salmon (In pieces)

2 tablespoons coconut oil

1 tablespoon tandoori seasoning

Ingredients for the Cucumber Sauce

½ cup shredded cucumber

1 ¼ cup sour cream or mayonnaise

2 minced garlic cloves

Juice of ½ of a lime

Optional: ½ teaspoon salt

Ingredients for the Crispy Salad

3 ½ ounces arugula lettuce

3 scallions

1 yellow pepper

Juice of 1 lime

2 avocados

Instructions

1. Preheat the oven to 350°F.

2. Mix the tandoori seasoning and the 2 tablespoons of oil to coat the salmon.

3. Bake the salmon for fifteen to twenty minutes.

4. Combine the lime juice, garlic, cucumber (blot the water out with paper towels first), and sour cream/mayonnaise in a mixing dish.

5. Prepare the salad ingredients and enjoy.

Yields: Four Servings

Dinner: Ground Beef Stir Fry

Ingredients

300 g (approximately 10 ½ ounces) ground beef

5 medium brown mushrooms

½ cup broccoli

2 leaves kale

½ medium Spanish onion

1 Tbsp. coconut oil

½ medium red pepper

1 Tbsp. cayenne pepper

1 Tbsp. Chinese Five Spices

Note: McCormick was used for the Five Spices

Instructions

1. Prepare the vegetables—slice the mushrooms—chop the broccoli.

2. Heat a frying pan on the stovetop using the med-high setting. Pour in the oil and toss in the onions. Cook for an additional minute.

3. Blend the remainder of the vegetables and cook an additional two minutes—stirring often.

4. Combine the spices and beef—lower the heat to medium—and continue cooking for approximately two more minutes.

5. Cover the pan and cook for five or ten more minutes until the beef is done.

Serving Portion: 1 (Recipe is for three servings): Fat: 18 g; Carbs 7 g; Protein: 29 g; Calories: 307

Day 9

Breakfast: Cheddar and Sage Waffles

Ingredients

1 1/3 coconut flour

1 teaspoon ground sage

½ teaspoon salt

¼ teaspoon garlic powder

3 teaspoons baking powder

2 cups canned coconut milk

½ cup water

3 tablespoons melted coconut oil

1 cup shredded cheddar cheese

2 eggs

Instructions

1. Prepare the waffle iron on the required manufacturer's setting. Grease the iron (top and bottom).

2. Blend all of the seasonings, flour, and baking powder in a container.

3. Mix the wet ingredients, stirring until the batter becomes stiff. Blend in the cheese.

4. Scoop out a one-third cup of the batter and place in each section of the iron.

5. Depending on how you like your waffles; you can run them through two cycles on the iron if you want it crispier.

Serving Portion: 1 waffles (The recipe serves 12): Fat: 17.21 g; Carbs 9.2 g; Protein: 6.52 g; Calories: 213.97

Lunch: Crispy Shrimp Salad on an Egg Wrap

Ingredients for the Wraps

1-ounce butter

4 eggs

Pepper and salt to taste

Shrimp Salad Ingredients

6 ounces shrimp

2 avocados

1/2 of an apple/handful of radishes

1 teaspoon lime juice

1 celery stalk

1 cup mayonnaise

1 red chili pepper

8 tablespoons fresh parsley or cilantro

Instructions for the Wrap

1. Cook and peel the shrimp. Finely chop the red chili pepper and fresh cilantro/parsley.

2. Whip the eggs with the pepper and salt.

3. Using a medium frying pan, melt the butter. Empty half of the egg batter until the egg gets firm, and repeat for the second one.

Instructions for the Salad

1. Slice the avocado and scoop out providing you with ½-inch cubes. Place them in a dish and give a fresh squeeze of juice over them and mix.

2. Dice the apple and thinly slice the celery, putting them with the avocado. Blend in the peppers, cilantro/parsley, and mayonnaise.

3. Combine well and gently stir in the shrimps. Add more salt if desired.

Yields: Two Servings

This is one of those meals that can be enjoyed with leafy greens or alone. Add a couple of boiled eggs in place of the wrap for another healthy choice.

Dinner: Bacon Wrapped Meatloaf

Ingredients

1 finely chopped yellow onion

1 ½ Pounds ground lamb, poultry, pork *or* beef

2 tablespoons butter

8 tablespoons heavy whipping cream

1 egg

6 ¾ tablespoons shredded cheese

1 tablespoon dried basil/oregano

1 tsp. salt

½ tsp. black pepper

7 ¾ ounces sliced bacon

Optional: ½ tablespoon tamari soy sauce

For the Gravy: 1 ¼ cups heavy whipping cream

Instructions

1. Preheat the oven to 400°F/200°C.

2. Saute the onion in a pan with the butter, but don't brown it.

3. Combine the meat in a container, adding all of the remainders of ingredients but omit the bacon. Don't over-work it, but blend the ingredients well, making a loaf.

4. Bake it in the center of the oven for approximately 45 minutes. You can use some aluminum foil to cover the meatloaf, just in case, the bacon begins to scorch.

5. Reserve any of the accumulated juices and make the gravy, blending it with the cream in a small saucepan.

6. Let the mixture come to a boil using low heat until it is creamy and the right texture, usually for approximately ten to fifteen minutes.

7. Spice it up with a drizzle of tamari soy sauce for a bit of flavor.

8. Have some cauliflower or broccoli on the side with some butter. It is all up to you to decide on the veggie choices.

Yields: Four Servings

Day 10

Breakfast: Omelet Wrap with Avocado & Salmon

Ingredients

3 large eggs

½ package smoked salmon (100 g or 1.8 ounces)

½ avocado (3.5 ounces or 100 g)

1 spring onion (1/2 ounce or 15 g)

2 tablespoons cream cheese (full-fat—2.3 ounces or 64 g)

2 tablespoons chives (freshly chopped)

1 tablespoon butter or ghee

Instructions

1. In a mixing bowl—add a pinch of pepper and salt along with the eggs. Use a fork or whisk—mixing them well. Blend the chives and cream cheese.

2. Prepare the salmon and avocado (peel and slice).

3. In a sauté pan, melt the butter/ghee, and add the egg mixture. Cook until fluffy.

4. Put the omelet on a serving dish, and spoon the mixture of cheese over it.

5. Sprinkle the onion, prepared avocado, and salmon into the wrap.

Close and enjoy!

Serving Portion: Fat: 66.9g; Carbs 13.3 g; Protein: 36.9 g

Lunch: Tuna Avocado Melt

Ingredients

1-10 - ounce can drained tuna

1 medium cubed avocado

¼ cup mayonnaise

1/3 cup almond flour

¼ teaspoon onion powder

¼ cup parmesan cheese

½ teaspoon garlic powder

1/2 cup coconut oil (for frying)

Instructions

1. In a mixing container, blend all of the ingredients except for the coconut oil and avocado. Fold the cubed avocado into the tuna.

2. Make balls and coat each one with the almond flour.

3. Use the medium heat setting and put the oil in a pan—mix the tuna—and continue cooking until brown.

Note: Some people like to use this as a casserole dish.

Yields: Twelve Servings

Per Serving Portion: Fat: 11.8 g; Carbs 2.0 g; Protein: 6.2 g; Calories: 134.7

Dinner: Hamburger Patties with Fried Cabbage

Ingredients for the Hamburger Patties

1 egg

1 ½ Pounds ground beef

3 ¼ ounces feta cheese

1 tsp. salt

¼ tsp. ground black pepper

1 ¾ ounces finely- chopped, fresh parsley

1-ounce butter

1 tablespoon olive oil

Ingredients for the Gravy

1 ¾ - Ounces fresh (coarsely chopped) parsley

1 ¼ cups heavy whipping cream

Pepper and Salt

2 tablespoons tomato paste

Ingredients for the Green Cabbage

4 ¼ ounces butter

1 ½ Pounds shredded green cabbage

Pepper and Salt

Instructions

1. Form eight oblong patties by blending all of the ingredients listed under the hamburger patties.

2. Using the med-high setting on the stovetop, prepare a skillet with olive oil and butter and fry the patties for a minimum of ten minutes.

3. Empty the whipping cream and tomato paste into the mixture—stir— and let them blend.

Serve with some parsley for garnishment.

Instructions for Butter-fried Green Cabbage

1. Use a food processor or knife to shred the cabbage.

2. Prepare a frying pan with the butter and sauté the cabbage for approximately fifteen minutes on the med-high setting.

3. Reduce the heat for the last five minutes (or so)—stirring regularly.

Variations: You can also enjoy this with whatever you desire, including spinach, carrots, mushrooms, acorn squash, or corn.

Yields: Four Servings

Day 11

Breakfast: The Breadless Breakfast Sandwich

Ingredients

4 Eggs

1-ounce ham/pastrami cold cuts

2 tablespoons butter

2 ounces of edam/provolone/cheddar cheese

Several drops of Worcestershire or Tabasco sauce

Pepper and salt to taste

Instructions

1. Cut the cheese into thick slices.

2. Prepare a frying pan over medium heat. Fry the eggs over-easy with a pinch of pepper and salt.

3. Add the choice of meat onto the two eggs, a layer of cheese, and the egg for the top of the 'bun.'

4. Give the sandwich a splash of Worcestershire sauce/Tabasco and serve. You can also use some French Dijon mustard to complement the ham.

Yields: Two Servings

Lunch: Thai Fish With Coconut & Curry

Ingredients

1 ½ Pounds whitefish/salmon

4 tablespoons butter/ghee

Pepper and salt

1 to 2 tablespoons green/red curry paste

8 tablespoons fresh chopped cilantro

1 can coconut cream

1 Pound broccoli/cauliflower

For Greasing the Dish: Olive oil/butter

Instructions

1. Grease a baking dish. Preheat the oven to 400°F.

2. Place the salmon/fish in a dish where there is not any extra space between the dish and fish (not meant as a rhyme).

3. Place a dab of butter on each piece along with a shake of pepper and salt.

4. Combine the chopped cilantro, curry paste and coconut cream in a small container. Pour it over the fish.

5. Bake until the fish is falling apart done, usually about twenty minutes.

6. Boil the broccoli/cauliflower in water (lightly salted) for several minutes as a side dish.

Yields: Four Servings

Dinner: Keto Tacos or Nachos

Ingredients

500 g or 17.6 ounces ground beef

1 medium white onion (3.0 ounces)

4 tacos

1 teaspoon chili powder

2 garlic cloves

½ teaspoon ground cumin

2 teaspoons extra-virgin coconut oil or ghee

1 tablespoon unsweetened tomato puree

1 cup water (8 ounces)

½ teaspoon salt—more or less

Cayenne pepper or freshly ground black pepper

Topping Ingredients

1 small head of lettuce (approximately 3.5 ounces or 100 g)

1 cup or 5.3 ounces cherry tomatoes

1 medium avocado (7.1 ounces or 200 g)

Optional Toppings

4 tablespoons sour cream

1 cup grated cheese

Veggies including cabbage, cucumbers, or peppers

Instructions

1. Using med-high, add some butter/ghee in a frying pan; toss in the onion. Sauté until brown and mix in the beef, continue cooking until the beef is done.

2. Add the cumin and chili powder. (You can substitute with 1 ½ teaspoon of paprika.)

3. Pour in the water and add the tomato puree. Also add pepper, and salt if you like for additional flavoring.

4. Continue cooking until the meat is done and approximately ¼ of the sauce is reduced. Set to the side and prepare the vegetable topping.

5. Use the meat mixture to stuff the shells. Garnish with some of the tomatoes, lettuce, and avocado.

6. As an option, you can add a bit of sour cream or cheddar cheese.

Note: You may use this as a tasty taco or on the side with the meat as the centerfold for the remainder of the veggies.

The choice is all yours!

Day 12

Breakfast: Scrambled Eggs With Halloumi Cheese

Ingredients

5 to 6 eggs

3 ½ ounces diced Halloumi cheese

4 ½ ounces diced bacon

8 tablespoons each:

- Pitted olives

- Chopped fresh parsley

Pepper and Salt to taste

2 scallions

2 tablespoons olive oil

Instructions

1. Dice the bacon and cheese.

2. Over the stovetop, use the medium-high setting; pour the oil into a frying pan. Add the scallions, cheese, and bacon—sauté until browned.

3. Whip/Whisk the eggs, pepper, salt, and parsley in a mixing container.

4. Pour the mixture into the pan over the cheese and bacon.

5. Reduce the heat—toss in the olives and sauté for several minutes.

6. All Ready! You can enjoy this with or without a salad.

Yields: Two Servings

Lunch: Salmon with Spinach and Chili Tones

Ingredients

1 tablespoon chili paste

1 ½ Pounds Salmon (in pieces)

1 cup sour cream/mayonnaise

1 ¾ cup olive oil/butter

1 Pound fresh spinach

4 tablespoons grated parmesan cheese

Pepper and Salt

Instructions

1. Place the oven setting to 400°F/200°C. Use some cooking oil to coat a baking dish/pan.

2. Flavor the salmon with the pepper and salt. Place in the dish skin side down.

3. Blend the chili paste, sour cream/mayonnaise, and parmesan cheese and spread it on the filets.

4. Bake until the salmon is done—usually fifteen to twenty minutes.

5. In the meantime, sauté the spinach until it wilts using the oil/butter.

Yields: Four Servings

Dinner: Chicken Stuffed Avocado—Cajun Style

Ingredients

1 ½ cups cooked chicken (7.4 ounces or 210 g)

2 medium or 1 large avocados (10.6 ounces or 300 g)

2 tablespoons cream cheese/sour cream

2 tablespoons lemon juice (fresh)

¼ cup mayonnaise

½ teaspoon each: onion powder & garlic powder

¼ teaspoon each: salt and cayenne pepper

1 teaspoon each: paprika and dried thyme

Instructions

1. Shred the chicken into small pieces.

2. Blend all of the ingredients—saving the salt and lemon juice until last.

3. Leave one-half to one-inch of the avocado flesh—scoop the middle. Remove the seeds.

4. Cut the center/scooped pieces of avocado into small pieces and fill each of the halves with the mixture of chicken.

Yields: Two Servings

Serving Portion: Fat: 50.6 g; Carbs 16.4 g; Protein: 34.5 g

Day 13

Breakfast: Western Omelet

Ingredients

2 tablespoons sour cream/heavy whipping cream

6 eggs

Pepper and Salt

2 ounces butter

3 ½ ounces shredded cheese

5 ounces of ham

½ each:

- Finely chopped green bell peppers

- Finely chopped yellow onion

Instructions

1. Whisk the sour cream/cream and eggs until fluffy. Flavor with the pepper and salt. Add half of the cheese and combine.

2. Melt the butter on the stovetop on the medium heat setting. Sauté the peppers, onions, and ham for just a few minutes.

3. Pour the batter in and fry until the omelet is almost firm.

4. Lower the heat and Sprinkle the remainder of the cheese on top of your masterpiece. Fold the omelet right away.

Have a fresh green salad as a perfect brunch touch!

Yields: Two Servings

Lunch: Tortilla Ground Beef Salsa

Ingredients

1 ½ Pounds ground lamb/beef

8 to 12 low-carb tortilla breads

2 tablespoons olive oil

1 cup of water

Tex-Mex seasoning (see below)

1 teaspoon salt

Shredded leafy greens

17 to 27 tablespoons shredded cheese

Salsa Ingredients

1 to 2 diced tomatoes

2 avocados

1 tablespoon olive oil

Juice of 1 lime

8 tablespoons fresh cilantro

Pepper and Salt

Tex-Mex Seasoning

2 tsp. each:

- Paprika powder

- Chili powder

1 to 2 tsp. garlic/onion powder

1 tsp. ground cumin

A pinch of cayenne pepper

Optional: 1 tsp. salt

Instructions

1. Prepare two batches of low-carb tortilla bread (see below).

2. Chop the cilantro. Take out the beef so it can become room temperature. Cold meats can have an effect on the cooking times, and it is more of a boil, not a fry.

3. On the stovetop, heat the oil using a large pan. Toss in the beef, and cook for around ten minutes.

4. Add the salt, water, and taco seasoning to the beef and simmer until most of the liquid has evaporated.

5. Meanwhile, prepare the salsa with all of the ingredients.

6. Serve on the tortilla bread with some shredded cheese along with the leafy greens.

Yields: Four Servings

Low-Carb Tortillas

Ingredients

2 egg whites

2 eggs

6 ounces cream cheese

1 tablespoon coconut flour

1 to 2 teaspoons ground psyllium husk powder

½ teaspoon salt

Instructions

1. Heat the oven to 400°F. Prepare two baking sheets with parchment paper.

2. Whip the eggs and whites until fluffy. Blend in the cream cheese and whisk until creamy.

3. Combine the coconut flour, psyllium powder, and salt in a small container. Add the flour mixture for the batter a spoon at a time.

4. Spread out the batter on the baking tins, spreading thin, about ¼-inch thick. You can make two rectangles or four to six circles.

5. Bake until the tortilla begins to brown around the edges, usually about five minutes (or so).

6. Serve with some of your *Tex-Mex Ground Beef and Salsa.*

Yields: Two Servings

Dinner: Fish Casserole with Mushrooms

Ingredients

1 Pound mushrooms

3 ¼ ounces butter

2 Tbsp. fresh parsley

1 t. salt

Pepper (to taste)

2 C. heavy whipping cream

2 tablespoons fresh parsley

2 to 3 Tbsp. Dijon mustard

1 ½ Pounds white fish (Ex. Cod)

½ Pound shredded cheese

1 1/3 pounds cauliflower/broccoli

3 ¼ ounces olive oil/butter

Instructions

1. Heat the oven to 350°F. Lightly grease a baking dish for the fish.

2. Slice the mushrooms into wedges. *Sauté* in a pan with the butter, pepper, salt, and other herbs.

3. Empty the mustard and cream into the mixture and reduce the heat. Simmer for five to ten minutes until the sauce thickens.

4. Flavor the fish with the pepper and salt and add it to the prepared container. Sprinkle with ¾ of the cheese. Pour the creamed mushroom mixture over it and the rest of the cheese as a topping.

5. Bake approximately thirty minutes if the fish are frozen (less if not). After 20 minutes, test the fish to see if it flakes apart easily. Remember, the fish will cook for several minutes after it is removed from the oven.

6. Prepare the cauliflower into small florets, removing the leaves and stalks. You can use the entire broccoli by cutting it into rods/lengthwise.

7. Boil the veggie of choice, drain and add some butter/olive oil.

8. Coarsely mash with a fork or wooden spoon; adding some pepper and salt, and serve with your fish.

Yields: Four Servings

Day 14

Breakfast: Blueberry Smoothie

Smoothie Ingredients

1 C. fresh or frozen blueberries

1 2/3 C. coconut milk

1 Tbsp. lemon juice

½ tsp. vanilla extract

Instructions

1. Put all of the ingredients into a tall beaker. Mix using a hand mixer.

2. Pour the lemon juice in for additional flavoring.

Notes: You can substitute 1 ¼ cups of Greek yogurt for a dairy option and adjust with a small amount of water if you are searching for more liquid consistency. Add 1 tablespoon of a healthy oil such as coconut for more satiety.

Yields: Two Servings

Lunch: Cheeseburger

Ingredients

7 ounces shredded cheese

1 ½ Pounds ground beef

2 teaspoons each:

- Onion powder

- Garlic powder

- Paprika

For Frying

2 tablespoons fresh oregano

Finely chopped butter

Salsa

2 scallions

2 tomatoes

1 avocado

Fresh Cilantro (to taste)

Salt

1 tablespoon olive oil

Toppings

- Lettuce

- Cooked bacon

- Dijon mustard

- Mayonnaise

- Pickled jalapenos

- Dill pickle

Instructions

1. Chop all of the salsa ingredients in a small container and set to the side.

2. Combine all of the seasonings and ½ of the cheese into the beef mixture.

3. Prepare four burgers and grill or pan fry to your liking—adding cheese at the end of the cooking cycle.

4. Serve on the bed of lettuce with some mustard and a dill pickle.

Yields: Four Servings

Dinner: Turkey with Cream Cheese Sauce

Ingredients

1 1/3 Pounds turkey breast

2 tablespoons butter

2 cups heavy whipping cream/sour cream

7 ounces cream cheese

Pepper and salt

1 tablespoon tamari soy sauce

6 ¾ tablespoons small capers

Instructions

1. Heat the oven to 350°F.

2. *Sprinkle the turkey with pepper and salt for seasoning.*

3. *Add the butter to a frying pan. Sauté the turkey until golden. Place in the oven to finish cooking.*

4. *Using a small pan, combine the heavy cream/sour cream and cream cheese, bringing it to a boil; lower the heat and cook slowly for a few minutes.*

5. *On high heat in a small pan, use a small amount of butter or oil to fry the capers or enjoy them fresh.*

6. *When the turkey breast and veggies are done, add the sauce and capers on top of the turkey and serve along with some side dishes such as cauliflower or broccoli.*

Yields: Four Servings

Chapter 3: Additional Breakfast Recipes

Chia Pudding

Ingredients

1 cup light coconut milk

¼ cup chia seeds

½ tablespoon light corn syrup

Instructions

1. Combine all of the ingredients in a small mason jar or bowl.

2. Refrigerate overnight. It is ready when the seeds have gelled, and the pudding is thick.

3. Add some nuts and fresh fruit and 'dive in.'

Cow-time Breakfast Skillet

Ingredients

2 medium diced sweet potatoes

1 Pound breakfast sausage

5 eggs

Handful of cilantro

1 diced avocado

Hot sauce

Optional: Raw cheese

Pepper and Salt

Instructions

1. Heat the oven to 400°F.

2. Use medium heat on the stovetop; place an iron or oven-safe skillet. Crumble and brown the sausage. Remove the sausage, cook the potatoes until crunchy, and reserve the grease.

3. Put the sausage back in the pan. Make some spaces in the 'wells' of the skillet, enough room for one egg. Crack the eggs into each of the wells.

4. Put the skillet into the preheated oven and bake enough for the eggs to set (about 5 minutes). Turn up the thermostat in the oven to the broil setting to let it broil the tops of the yolks with the crispy sweet potatoes.

5. Take the skillet out of the oven and cover it with some cilantro, avocado, and hot sauce.

Enjoy the tasty different flavors.

Cream Cheese Pancakes

Ingredients for the Pancakes

2 oz. (room temperature) cream cheese

2 organic eggs

½ teaspoon cinnamon

1 teaspoon granulated sugar substitute

Instructions

1. Place each of the pancake ingredients into a blender. Blend until creamy smooth; letting it rest for two minutes for the bubbles to settle back down.

2. Grease a pan with Pam spray or butter.

3. Pour about ¼ of the pancake batter into the hot pan; cooking for two minutes. Flip and continue cooking about one more minute.

4. Serve with berries or a sugar-free syrup of your choice.

*Yield*s: Four Pancakes

Serving Size: 1 Batch: Carbs 2.5 g net; Fat 29; Protein 17 g; Calories 344

Dairy-Free Latte

Ingredients

2 Tbsp. coconut oil

1 2/3 C. hot water

2 eggs

1 tsp. ground ginger/pumpkin pie spice

Splash of vanilla extract

Instructions

1. Use a stick blender to combine all of the ingredients.

2. If you want to replace the spices; you can use 1 tablespoon of instant coffee or cocoa.

Enjoy for a quick boost!

Yields: Two Servings

Keto Sausage Patties

Ingredients

1 teaspoon maple extract

2 tablespoons granular Swerve Sweetener

½ teaspoon pepper

1 pound ground pork

2 tablespoons sage (chopped fresh)

1/8 teaspoon cayenne

1 teaspoon salt

¼ teaspoon garlic powder

Instructions

1. Combine each of the ingredients in a large mixing container.

2. Shape the patties to about a one-inch thickness.

3. The recipe will make eight equal patties.

4. Add a small amount of olive oil or a dab of butter to a pan over medium heat. For each side, allow three to four minutes.

Serving Portion: 2 patties: Carbs 1.4 g; Fat: 11 g; Protein: 21 g; Calories: 187

Keto Bacon

Use the Regular Oven

1. Preheat to 350 °F.

2. Put the bacon on a baking tray. Bake 20 to 25 minutes

3. Drain on a paper towel.

Use the Microwave

1. Put the bacon on paper towels in a single layer on a microwave-safe dish.

2. Use the high setting for four to six minutes.

Use the Skillet

1. Prepare the pan on the medium-low to medium.

2. Put the bacon into the pan single-layered.

3. Cook until the desired doneness is acquired.

Serving Portion: 2 slices: Fat: 19 g; Carbs 0.0 g; Protein: 7 g; Calories: 200

Mushroom Omelet

Ingredients

3 eggs

7/8 ounces shredded cheese

2 to 3 mushrooms

Optional: 1/5 of an onion

Pepper and salt to taste

For frying: 7/8 ounces butter

Instructions

1. Whisk the eggs with the pepper and salt, add the spices.

2. On the stovetop, use a frying pan to melt the butter. Pour in the eggs.

3. When the omelet begins to cook to firmness; sprinkle the mushrooms, cheese, and onion on top.

4. Ease the edges up using a spatula, and fold in half. Remove from the pan when golden brown.

If you are having brunch; add a crispy salad.

Yields: One serving

Chapter 4: Additional Lunch and Dinner Recipes

Deviled Eggs

With this tasty combination; it is hard to say breakfast or lunch; maybe brunch!

Ingredients

6 large eggs

¼ teaspoon yellow mustard

1 tablespoon mayonnaise

1 teaspoon paprika

Garnish: Parsley/salt/pepper

Optional

- ½ teaspoon cayenne pepper

- Several drops hot sauce

- 1 teaspoon cumin

Instructions

1. Slice the eggs lengthwise.

2. Mix the egg yolks with the rest of the ingredients.

3. Put the goodies inside the egg bed.

4. Sprinkle with condiments as desired.

Serving Portion: Fat: 20 g; Carbs 1 g; Protein: 19 g; Calories: 265

Ham and Apple Flatbread

Crust Ingredients

¾ cup almond flour

2 cups grated mozzarella cheese (part-skim)

2 tablespoons cream cheese

1/8 teaspoon dried thyme

½ teaspoon sea salt

Topping Ingredients

4 ounces sliced ham (low-carb)

½ small red onion

1 cup grated Mexican cheese

¼ medium apple

1/8 teaspoon dried thyme

Instructions

1. Remove the seeds and core from the apples. You can leave them unpeeled but will need to use a vegetable peeler to make the thin slices.

2. Heat the oven to 425°F.

3. Cut two pieces of parchment paper to fit into a 12-inch pizza pan (approximately two inches larger than the pan).

4. Use the high-heat setting and place a double boiler (water in the bottom pan), and bring the water to boiling. Lower the heat setting and add the cream cheese, mozzarella cheese, salt, thyme, and almond flour to the top of the double boiler—stirring constantly.

5. When the cheese mixture resembles dough, place it on one of the pieces of parchment—and knead the dough until totally mixed.

6. Roll the dough into a ball—placing it at the center of the paper—place the second piece of paper over the top, and roll with a rolling pin (or a large glass).

7. Place the dough onto the pizza pan (leaving the paper connected).

8. Poke several holes in the dough and put into the preheated oven for approximately six to eight minutes.

9. When browned, remove it, and lower the setting of the oven to 350°F.

10. Arrange the cheese, apple slices, onion slices, and ham pieces.

11. Top off with the remainder (3/4 cup) of cheese.

12. Season with the ground pepper, salt, and thyme.

13. Place the finished product into the oven, baking until you see a golden brown crust.

14. Slide it from the parchment paper and cool two or three minutes before cutting.

Yields: Eight Slices

Tip: If you do not own a double boiler; you can substitute with a mixing dish over a pot of boiling water as a substitute.

Serving Portion: 1: Fat: 20 g; Carbs 5 g; Protein: 16 g; Calories: 255

Chicken Breast with Herb Butter

Ingredients for the Fried Chicken

4 Chicken Breasts

Pepper and Salt

1-ounce of olive oil/butter

Herb Butter Ingredients

1 clove garlic

1/3 Pound butter (room temperature)

1 tsp. lemon juice

½ tsp. each:

- garlic powder

- salt

4 Tbsp. fresh chopped parsley

Leafy Greens

½ Pound leafy greens (baby spinach for example)

Instructions

1. Take the butter out of the refrigerator for at least thirty to sixty minutes before you begin to prepare your meal.

2. Add all of the ingredients, including the butter, and blend thoroughly in a small container; set to the side.

3. Use the pepper and salt to flavor the chicken. Cook the chicken filets in a skillet using the butter over medium heat. To avoid dried out filets, lower the temperature the last few minutes.

4. Serve over a bed of greens with some melted herb butter over the top.

Yields: Four Servings

Low-Carbonara

Ingredients

2/3 Pounds diced Pancetta/bacon

1 ¼ cups heavy whipping cream

1 tablespoon butter

3 1/3 tablespoons mayonnaise

Fresh chopped parsley

Pepper and salt

2 Pounds zucchini

3 ½ ounces grated Parmesan cheese

4 egg yolks

Instructions

1. Empty the heavy cream into a saucepan, bringing it to a boil. Lower the burner and continue boiling until the juices are reduced by about a third.

2. Fry the bacon/pancetta; reserve the fat.

3. Combine the heavy cream, mayonnaise, pepper, and salt into the saucepan mixture.

4. Make 'zoodles' out of the zucchini using a potato peeler or spiralizer.

5. Add the zoodles to the warm sauce and serve with egg yolks, bacon, parsley, and freshly grated cheese.

6. Drizzle a bit of the bacon grease on top.

Yummy!

Yields: Four Servings

Pesto Chicken Casserole with Olives and Cheese

Ingredients

1 ½ Pounds chicken breasts/thighs

3 ½ ounces green or red pesto

8 tablespoons pitted olives

1 2/3 cups heavy whipping cream

½ Pound diced feta cheese

Pepper and Salt

1 finely chopped garlic clove

For Frying: Butter

For Serving

- Olive oil

- 1/3 Pound leafy greens

- Sea salt

Instructions

1. Heat the oven to 400°F.

2. Cut the chicken into pieces and flavor with the pepper and salt.

3. Place in a skillet with the butter, cooking until well done.

4. Combine the heavy cream and pesto.

5. Put the chicken pieces in the baking dish with the garlic, feta cheese, and olives, along with the pesto mix.

6. Bake for 20 to 30 minutes until the perfect color.

Enjoy with some green beans, sautéed asparagus, or another veggie of your choice.

Yields: Four Servings

Red Pesto Pork Chops

Ingredients

4 Pork chops

4 tablespoons red pesto

2 tablespoons olive oil/butter

6 tablespoons mayonnaise

Instructions

1. Thoroughly rub the chops with the pesto.

2. Fry on medium heat in a skillet with oil/butter for eight minutes. Reduce the heat and simmer four more minutes.

3. Serve with the pesto mayonnaise: 6 tablespoons of mayonnaise (+) 1 to 2 tablespoons pesto.

Serve with a large salad. You can also add a serving of cauliflower and broccoli with cheese.

Chapter 5:

Snacks and Desserts for the Diet Plan

Keto Ginger Snap Cookies

Ingredients

¼ cup unsalted butter

1 large egg

2 C. almond flour

½ tsp. ground cinnamon

1 tsp. vanilla extract

1 C. sugar substitute/Erythritol (Swerve)

2 tsp. ground ginger

¼ tsp. each:

- Salt
- Ground cloves
- Nutmeg

Instructions

1. Set the oven to 350°F.
2. Combine the dry ingredients in a small dish.
3. Combine the remainder components to the dry mixture, and mix using a hand blender/mixer. (The dough will be crumbly and stiff.)
4. Measure out the dough for each cookie and flatten with a fork or your fingers.
5. Bake for approximately nine to eleven minutes or till they are browned.

Yields: 24 Cookies

Pumpkin Pudding

Ingredients

¼ cup pumpkin puree

1/3 cup granulated (Erythritol/Stevia)

½ tsp. pumpkin pie spices

1 tsp. xanthan gum

3 medium egg yolks

1 ½ cups whipping cream

1 tsp. vanilla extract

For the Cream Mixture

3 Tbsp. granulated stevia

1 cup whipping cream

½ tsp. vanilla extract

Instructions

1. Blend the pumpkin spice, xanthan gum, sweetener, and salt. Whip/whisk until the texture is smooth. Add the yolks, puree, and vanilla extract to the mixture; blend thoroughly.

2. Slowly pour in the whipping cream, after all of the cream is added. Using medium heat let the mixture come to a boil.

3. Continue the process for about 4 to 7 minutes, until thickened.

4. Place in the refrigerator in a container. Stir every ten minutes.

5. Meanwhile, in a medium dish, use a mixer to whip the one cup of whipping cream resulting in stiff peaks. Add the vanilla and sweetener; stir gently.

6. After the base pudding mixture has cooled; fold the whipped cream into the mix.

Scoop the pudding into small serving dishes and chill for a minimum of one to two hours.

Note: The Xanthan gum is available on Amazon.

Yields: Six Servings

No-Bake Cashew Coconut Bars

Ingredients

¼ cup maple syrup/sugar-free

1 cup almond flour

¼ cup melted butter

1 teaspoon cinnamon

½ cup cashews

A pinch of salt

1/4 cup shredded coconut

Instructions

1. Combine the flour and melted butter in a large mixing dish.

2. Add the maple syrup, cinnamon, salt, and coconut—blend well.

3. Use roasted or raw cashews. Chop them and add to the cashew-coconut bar dough. Blend well again.

4. Cover a cookie pan with parchment paper and spread the dough onto the paper in an even layer.

5. Place in the fridge for a minimum of two hours. Slice them and enjoy!

Yields: Eight Servings

Brownie Cheesecake

The Brownie Base Ingredients:

2 ounces chopped unsweetened chocolate

2 large eggs

½ cup butter

1/2 cup almond flour

1 pinch of salt

¼ cup cocoa powder

¾ cup granulated Erythritol/Swerve Sweetener

¼ cup pecans/walnuts (chopped)

¼ teaspoon vanilla

Cheesecake Filling Ingredients

2 large eggs

1 pound softened cream cheese

½ cup granulated sugar/Swerve sweetener

½ teaspoon vanilla extract

¼ cup heavy cream

Instructions

1. Butter a nine-inch springform pan; wrapping the bottom with foil.

2. Set the oven at 325°F.

3. Melt the chocolate and butter in a microwave-safe dish for 30 seconds.

4. Whisk the cocoa powder, almond flour, and salt in a small dish.

5. In a separate dish; whip the vanilla, eggs, and Swerve until smooth.

6. Blend the flour mixture and chocolate/butter mixture. Blend in the nuts.

7. Spread out in the prepared dish and bake for approximately 15 to 20 minutes.

8. Let it cool for about 20 to 25 minutes.

For the Filling

1. Reduce the oven setting to 300°F.

2. Blend the Swerve, the vanilla, cream, eggs, and cream cheese in a mixing container until everything is thoroughly mixed. Empty the filling ingredients into the crust and place it on a large cookie sheet.

3. Bake for about 35 to 45 minutes. The center should barely jiggle.

4. Loosen the edges with a knife.

5. Place them in the fridge for a minimum of three hours.

Yields: Ten Servings

Chocolate Soufflé

Ingredients

1/3 cup sugar substitute (Lakanto Mont Fruit/Amazon)

1 tablespoon butter

6 large egg whites

3 large egg yolks

5 ounces unsweetened chocolate

Note: The eggs work best at room temperature.

Instructions

1. Preset the oven to 375°F.

2. Use the butter to grease a soufflé dish.

3. Use a double boiler or a metal dish above a pan of boiling water to melt the chocolate. (Stir the mix constantly.)

4. Remove the dish and whip in the yolks until the mix hardens. Set it to the side.

5. Use a pinch of salt, whip/whisk the egg whites with an electric mixer on the highest setting.

6. Gradually, blend in the sugar/Lakanto. Continue until you see stiff peaks.

7. Stir in one cup of the egg whites into the chocolate combination folding gently using a silicone spatula. Pour the mixture into the soufflé dish.

8. Bake approximately twenty minutes. The center should still jiggle with

the soufflé crusted and puffed on the top.

Serve this delicious treat right away.

Topping/Optional: Coconut whipped cream

Yields: Four Treats

Note: To make the soufflé rise evenly; use your thumb to remove the batter from the top of the dish.

Macaroon Keto Bombs

Your curiosity is wondering, "What is a bomb?" The reasoning is that this is good for you and is too delicious to pass by when you are craving a treat!

Ingredients

½ cup shredded coconut

¼ cup almond flour

2 tablespoons sugar substitute (Swerve)

3 egg whites

1 tablespoon each:

- Coconut oil

- Vanilla extract

Instructions

1. Set the oven at 400°F.

2. In a small container, combine the almond flour, coconut, and Swerve.

3. Use a small saucepan to melt the coconut oil. Add the vanilla extract.

4. *Note*: To mount the egg whites, place a medium dish in the freezer.

5. Add the oil to the flour mixture and blend well.

6. Break the egg whites in the cold dish and whip until stiff peaks are formed. Blend the egg whites into the flour mixture.

7. Spoon the mixture into a muffin cup or place them on a baking sheet.

8. Bake the macaroons for eight minutes or until you see browned edges.

9. Cool the bombs before you attempt to remove them from the pan.

Yields: Ten Servings

Conclusion

Thank for viewing your personal copy of the *Ketogenic Diet: Better Energy, Performance, and Natural Fuel to Good Health for the Smart*. Let's hope it was informative and able to provide you with all of the tools you need to achieve your goals as a better energy management specialist.

The next step is to test some of the recipes for yourself and discover what you have been missing since you have tried so many times unsuccessfully using other dieting methods. The recipes provided have been tested by qualified chefs who know the deal when it comes to energy performance.

Just remember, making advances towards a better lifestyle begins at the breakfast, lunch, and dinner table. You can supplement as you see fit once you have the knack of how the balance works.

Index for Recipes

Chapter 2: The 14-Day Plan

Day One

- Breakfast: Keto Scrambled Eggs

- Lunch: Tuna Cheese Melt (Low-Carbs)

- "Oopsie" Bread

- Dinner: Chicken Smothered in Creamy Onion Sauce

Day Two

- Breakfast: Mock Mc Griddle Casserole

- Brussels Sprouts with Hamburger Gratin

- Dinner: Squash and Sausage Casserole

Day Three

- Breakfast: Can't Beat it Porridge

- Lunch: Salad From a Jar

- Dinner: Ham and Cheese Stromboli

Day Four

- Breakfast: Frittata with Cheese and Tomatoes

- Lunch: Chicken—Broccoli—Zucchini Boats

- Dinner: Steak-Lovers Slow-Cooked Chili

Day 5

- Breakfast: Brownie Muffins

- Lunch: Bacon-Avocado-Goat Cheese Salad

- Dinner: Tenderloin Stuffed Keto Style

Day 6

- Breakfast: Sausage—Feta—Spinach Omelet

- Lunch: Pancakes with Cream-Cheese Topping

- Dinner: Skillet Style Sausage and Cabbage Melt

Day 7

- Breakfast: Tapas

- Lunch: Tofu—Bok-Choy Salad

- Dinner: Hamburger Stroganoff

Day 8

- Breakfast: Cheddar—Jalapeno Waffles

- Lunch: Salmon Tandoori with Cucumber Sauce

- Dinner: Ground Beef Stir Fry

Day 9

- Breakfast: Cheddar and Sage Waffles

- Lunch: Crispy Shrimp Salad on an Egg Wrap

- Dinner: Bacon Wrapped Meatloaf

Day 10

- Breakfast: Omelet Wrap with Avocado & Salmon

- Lunch: Tuna Avocado Melt

- Dinner: Hamburger Patties with Fried Cabbage

Day 11

- Breakfast: The Breadless Breakfast Sandwich

- Lunch: Thai Fish With Coconut & Curry

- Dinner: Keto Tacos or Nachos

Day 12

- Breakfast: Scrambled Eggs With Halloumi Cheese

- Lunch: Salmon with Spinach and Chili Tones

- Dinner: Chicken Stuffed Avocado—Cajun Style

Day 13

- Breakfast: Western Omelet

- Lunch: Tortilla Ground Beef Salsa

- Low-Carb Tortillas

- Dinner: Fish Casserole with Mushrooms

Day 14

- Breakfast: Blueberry Smoothie

- Lunch: Cheeseburger

- Dinner: Turkey with Cream Cheese Sauce

Chapter 3: Additional Breakfast Recipes

- Chia Pudding

- Cow-time Breakfast Skillet

- Cream Cheese Pancakes

- Dairy Free Latte

- Keto Sausage Patties

- Keto Bacon

- Mushroom Omelet

Chapter 4: Additional Lunch and Dinner Recipes

- Deviled Eggs

- Ham and Apple Flatbread

- Chicken Breast with Herb Butter

- Low-Carbonara

- Pesto Chicken Casserole with Olives and Cheese

- Red Pesto Pork Chops

Chapter 5: Snacks and Desserts for the Diet Plan

- Keto Ginger Snap Cookies

- Pumpkin Pudding

- No-Bake Cashew Coconut Bars

- Brownie Cheesecake

- Chocolate Soufflé

Macaroon Keto Bombs

PART II

Chapter 1: Meal Planning 101

Sticking to a diet is something that is not the easiest in the world. When it comes down to it, we struggle to change up our diets on a whim. It might be that for the first few days, you are able to stick to it and make sure that you are only eating those foods that are better for you, but over time, you will get to a point where you feel the pressure to cave in. You might realize that sticking to your diet is difficult and think that stopping for a burger on your way home won't be too bad. You might think that figuring out lunch or dinner is too much of a hassle, or you realize that the foods that you have bought forgot a key ingredient that you needed for dinner.

The good news is, you have an easy fix. When you are able to figure out what you are making for yourself for your meals well in advance, you stop having to worry so much about the foods that you eat, what you do with them, and what you are going to reach for when it's time to eat. You will be able to change up what you are doing so that you can be certain that the meals that you are enjoying are good for you, and you won't have to worry so much about the stress that goes into it. Let's take a look at what you need to do to get started with meal planning so that you can begin to do so without having to think too much about it.

Make a Menu

First, before you do anything, make sure that you make a menu! This should be something that you do on your own, or you should sit down with your family to ask them what they prefer. If you can do this, you will be able to ensure that you've got a clear-cut plan. When you have a menu a week in advance, you save yourself time and money because you know that all of your meals will use ingredients that are similar, and you won't have to spend forever thinking about what you should make at any point in time.

Plan around Ads

When you do your menu, make it a point to glance through the weekly ads as well. Typically, you will find that there are plenty of deals that you can make use of that will save you money.

Go Meatless Once Per Week

A great thing to do that is highly recommended on the Mediterranean Diet is to have a day each week where you go meatless for dinner. By doing so, you will realize that you can actually cut costs and enjoy the foods more at the same time. It is a great way to get that additional fruit and veggie content into your day, and there are plenty of healthy options that are out there for you. You just have to commit to doing so. In the meal plans that you'll see below, you will notice that there will be a meatless day on Day 2 every week.

Use Ingredients That You Already Have On Hand

Make it a point to use ingredients that you already have on hand whenever possible. Alternatively, make sure that all of the meals that you eat during the week use very similar ingredients. When you do this, you know that you're avoiding causing any waste or losing ingredients along the way, meaning that you can save money. The good news is, on the Mediterranean diet, there are plenty of delicious meals that enjoy very similar ingredients that you can eat.

Avoid Recipes that Call for a Special Ingredient

If you're trying to avoid waste, it is a good idea for you to avoid any ingredients in meals that are not going to carry over to other meals during your weekly plan.

By avoiding doing so, you can usually save yourself that money for that one ingredient that would be wasted. Alternatively, if you find that you really want that dish, try seeing if you can freeze some of it for later. When you do that, you can usually ensure that your special ingredient at least didn't go to waste.

Use Seasonal Foods

Fruits and veggies are usually cheaper when you buy them in season, and even better, when you do so, you will be enjoying a basic factor of the Mediterranean diet just by virtue of enjoying the foods when they are fresh. Fresher foods are usually tastier, and they also tend to carry more vitamins and minerals because they have not had the chance to degrade over time.

Make Use of Leftovers and Extra Portions

One of the greatest things that you can do when it comes to meal planning is to make use of your leftovers and make-ahead meals. When you do this regularly, making larger portions than you need, you can then use the extras as lunches and dinners all week long, meaning that you won't have to be constantly worrying about the food that you eat for lunch. We will use some of these in the meal plans that you will see as well.

Eat What You Enjoy

Finally, the last thing to remember with your meal plan is that you ought to be enjoying the foods that are on it at all times. When you ensure that the foods that you have on your plate are those that you actually enjoy, sticking to your meal plan doesn't become such a chore, and that means that you will be able to do better as well with your own diet. Your meal plan should be loaded up with foods that you are actually excited about enjoying. Meal planning and dieting should not be a drag—you should love every moment of it!

Chapter 2: 1 Month Meal Plan

Week 1: Success is no accident—you have to reach for it

Day 1: Prep Day

Breakfast: Savory Mediterranean Breakfast Muffins *Reserve extras for week's breakfasts*

Lunch: Aglio e Olio and Broccoli

Dinner: Slow Cooker Vegetarian Mediterranean Stew *Double recipe and reserve extras for week's lunches*

Day 2

Breakfast: Savory Mediterranean Breakfast Muffins

Lunch: Slow Cooker Vegetarian Mediterranean Stew

Dinner: Vegetarian Toss Together Mediterranean Pasta Salad

Day 3

Breakfast: Savory Mediterranean Breakfast Muffins

Lunch: Slow Cooker Vegetarian Mediterranean Stew

Dinner: Cilantro and Garlic Baked Salmon

Day 4

Breakfast: Savory Mediterranean Breakfast Muffins

Lunch: Slow Cooker Vegetarian Mediterranean Stew

Dinner: Mediterranean Mahi Mahi

Day 5

Breakfast: Savory Mediterranean Breakfast Muffins

Lunch: Slow Cooker Vegetarian Mediterranean Stew

Dinner: Grilled Chicken Mediterranean Salad

Day 6

Breakfast: Greek Yogurt Parfait

Lunch: Harissa Pasta

Dinner: Spaghetti and Clams

Day 7

Breakfast: Apple Whipped Yogurt

Lunch: Leftover Spaghetti and Clams

Dinner: Lemon Herb Chicken and Potatoes One Pot meal

Week 2: Self-belief and effort will take you to what you want to achieve

Day 1: Prep Day

Breakfast: Make-Ahead Overnight Oats: *Set up a new jar every night before bed to have breakfast ready the next day. Change up toppings/fruits if you want some variety.*

Lunch: Chicken and Couscous Mediterranean Wraps

Dinner: Slow Cooker Chicken and Chickpea Soup: *Double the batch and take to work for the week for lunches*

Day 2

Breakfast: Make-Ahead Overnight Oats

Lunch: Slow Cooker Chicken and Chickpea Soup

Dinner: Vegetarian Greek Stuffed Mushrooms

Day 3

Breakfast: Make-Ahead Overnight Oats

Lunch: Slow Cooker Chicken and Chickpea Soup

Dinner: Sheet Pan Shrimp

Day 4

Breakfast: Make-Ahead Overnight Oats

Lunch: Slow Cooker Chicken and Chickpea Soup

Dinner: Slow Cooker Brisket: *Prepare this before work and set to low heat.*

Day 5

Breakfast: Make-Ahead Overnight Oats

Lunch: Slow Cooker Chicken and Chickpea Soup

Dinner: Grilled Chicken Mediterranean Salad

Day 6

Breakfast: Make-Ahead Overnight Oats

Lunch: Slow Cooker Chicken and Chickpea Soup

Dinner: Slow Cooker Mediterranean Chicken

Day 7

Breakfast: Make-Ahead Overnight Oats

Lunch: Mediterranean Feta Mac and Cheese

Dinner: Herbed Lamb and Veggies

Week 3: The harder you work, the greater the success

Day 1: Prep Day

Breakfast: Mediterranean Pastry Pinwheels: *These can be frozen before they are baked and then baked individually for 10-15 minutes in a toaster oven for an easy weekday breakfast. Prepare on Sunday and reserve some for on-the-go breakfasts for the week.*

Lunch: Vegetarian Mediterranean Quiche

Dinner: Moroccan Lentil Soup: *Double this recipe and use extras for lunch for the week.*

Day 2

Breakfast: Mediterranean Pastry Pinwheels

Lunch: Moroccan Lentil Soup

Dinner: Vegetarian Zucchini Lasagna Rolls

Day 3

Breakfast: Mediterranean Pastry Pinwheels

Lunch: Moroccan Lentil Soup

Dinner: Vegan Mediterranean Buddha Bowl

Day 4

Breakfast: Mediterranean Pastry Pinwheels

Lunch: Moroccan Lentil Soup

Dinner: Lemon Herb Chicken and Potatoes One Pot Meal

Day 5

Breakfast: Mediterranean Pastry Pinwheels

Lunch: Moroccan Lentil Soup

Dinner: Chicken and Couscous Mediterranean Wrap

Day 6

Breakfast: Mediterranean Pastry Pinwheels

Lunch: Moroccan Lentil Soup

Dinner: Cilantro and Garlic Baked Salmon

Day 7

Breakfast: Mediterranean Pastry Pinwheels

Lunch: Vegan Mediterranean Pasta

Dinner: Walnut Crusted Salmon with Rosemary

Week 4: You don't need perfection—you need effort

Day 1: Prep Day

Breakfast: Vegetarian Breakfast Sandwich

Lunch: Baked Feta with Olive Tapenade

Dinner: Vegetarian Slow Cooker Quinoa: *Double and use for lunches for the week.*

Day 2

Breakfast: Vegan Breakfast Toast

Lunch: Vegetarian Slow Cooker Quinoa

Dinner: Vegetarian Cheesy Artichoke and Spinach Stuffed Squash

Day 3

Breakfast: Vegan Breakfast Toast

Lunch: Vegetarian Slow Cooker Quinoa

Dinner: Herbed Lamb and Veggies

Day 4

Breakfast: Vegetarian Breakfast Sandwich

Lunch: Vegetarian Slow Cooker Quinoa

Dinner: slow-cooked Chicken and Chickpea Soup: *Double recipe and use for lunches for the rest of the week.*

Day 5

Breakfast: Vegetarian Breakfast Sandwich

Lunch: slow-cooked Chicken and Chickpea Soup

Dinner: Chickpea Stew

Day 6

Breakfast: Vegan Breakfast Toast

Lunch: slow-cooked Chicken and Chickpea Soup

Dinner: Garlic-Roasted Salmon with Brussels Sprouts

Day 7

Breakfast: Vegan Breakfast Toast

Lunch: slow-cooked Chicken and Chickpea Soup

Dinner: Mediterranean Cod

Chapter 3: 8 Week Meal Plan for Weight Loss

Week 1: Transformation happens one day at a time

Day 1: Prep Day

Breakfast: Savory Mediterranean Breakfast Muffins *Reserve extras for week's breakfasts*

Lunch: Aglio e Olio and Broccoli

Dinner: Slow Cooker Vegetarian Mediterranean Stew *Double recipe and reserve extras for week's lunches*

Day 2

Breakfast: Savory Mediterranean Breakfast Muffins

Lunch: Slow Cooker Vegetarian Mediterranean Stew

Dinner: Vegetarian Toss Together Mediterranean Pasta Salad

Day 3

Breakfast: Savory Mediterranean Breakfast Muffins

Lunch: Slow Cooker Vegetarian Mediterranean Stew

Dinner: Cilantro and Garlic Baked Salmon

Day 4

Breakfast: Savory Mediterranean Breakfast Muffins

Lunch: Slow Cooker Vegetarian Mediterranean Stew

Dinner: Mediterranean Mahi Mahi

Day 5

Breakfast: Savory Mediterranean Breakfast Muffins

Lunch: Slow Cooker Vegetarian Mediterranean Stew

Dinner: Grilled Chicken Mediterranean Salad

Day 6

Breakfast: Greek Yogurt Parfait

Lunch: Harissa Pasta

Dinner: Spaghetti and Clams

Day 7

Breakfast: Apple Whipped Yogurt

Lunch: Leftover Spaghetti and Clams

Dinner: Lemon Herb Chicken and Potatoes One Pot meal

Week 2: Success doesn't come to you—you go to it

Day 1: Prep Day

Breakfast: Make-Ahead Overnight Oats: *Set up a new jar every night before bed to have breakfast ready the next day. Change up toppings/fruits if you want some variety.*

Lunch: Chicken and Couscous Mediterranean Wraps

Dinner: Slow Cooker Chicken and Chickpea Soup: *Double the batch and take to work for the week for lunches*

Day 2

Breakfast: Make-Ahead Overnight Oats

Lunch: Slow Cooker Chicken and Chickpea Soup

Dinner: Vegetarian Greek Stuffed Mushrooms

Day 3

Breakfast: Make-Ahead Overnight Oats

Lunch: Slow Cooker Chicken and Chickpea Soup

Dinner: Sheet Pan Shrimp

Day 4

Breakfast: Make-Ahead Overnight Oats

Lunch: Slow Cooker Chicken and Chickpea Soup

Dinner: Slow Cooker Brisket: *Prepare this before work and set to low heat.*

Day 5

Breakfast: Make-Ahead Overnight Oats

Lunch: Slow Cooker Chicken and Chickpea Soup

Dinner: Grilled Chicken Mediterranean Salad

Day 6

Breakfast: Make-Ahead Overnight Oats

Lunch: Slow Cooker Chicken and Chickpea Soup

Dinner: Slow Cooker Mediterranean Chicken

Day 7

Breakfast: Make-Ahead Overnight Oats

Lunch: Mediterranean Feta Mac and Cheese

Dinner: Herbed Lamb and Veggies

Week 3: Success is about consistency

Day 1: Prep Day

Breakfast: Mediterranean Pastry Pinwheels: *These can be frozen before they are baked and then baked individually for 10-15 minutes in a toaster oven for an easy weekday breakfast. Prepare on Sunday and reserve some for on-the-go breakfasts for the week.*

Lunch: Vegetarian Mediterranean Quiche

Dinner: Moroccan Lentil Soup: *Double this recipe and use extras for lunch for the week.*

Day 2

Breakfast: Mediterranean Pastry Pinwheels

Lunch: Moroccan Lentil Soup

Dinner: Vegetarian Zucchini Lasagna Rolls

Day 3

Breakfast: Mediterranean Pastry Pinwheels

Lunch: Moroccan Lentil Soup

Dinner: Vegan Mediterranean Buddha Bowl

Day 4

Breakfast: Mediterranean Pastry Pinwheels

Lunch: Moroccan Lentil Soup

Dinner: Lemon Herb Chicken and Potatoes One Pot Meal

Day 5

Breakfast: Mediterranean Pastry Pinwheels

Lunch: Moroccan Lentil Soup

Dinner: Chicken and Couscous Mediterranean Wrap

Day 6

Breakfast: Mediterranean Pastry Pinwheels

Lunch: Moroccan Lentil Soup

Dinner: Cilantro and Garlic Baked Salmon

Day 7

Breakfast: Mediterranean Pastry Pinwheels

Lunch: Vegan Mediterranean Pasta

Dinner: Walnut Crusted Salmon with Rosemary

Week 4: Success is a journey

Day 1: Prep Day

Breakfast: Vegetarian Breakfast Sandwich

Lunch: Baked Feta with Olive Tapenade

Dinner: Vegetarian Slow Cooker Quinoa: *Double and use for lunches for the week.*

Day 2

Breakfast: Vegan Breakfast Toast

Lunch: Vegetarian Slow Cooker Quinoa

Dinner: Vegetarian Cheesy Artichoke and Spinach Stuffed Squash

Day 3

Breakfast: Vegan Breakfast Toast

Lunch: Vegetarian Slow Cooker Quinoa

Dinner: Herbed Lamb and Veggies

Day 4

Breakfast: Vegetarian Breakfast Sandwich

Lunch: Vegetarian Slow Cooker Quinoa

Dinner: slow-cooked Chicken and Chickpea Soup: *Double recipe and use for lunches for the rest of the week.*

Day 5

Breakfast: Vegetarian Breakfast Sandwich

Lunch: slow-cooked Chicken and Chickpea Soup

Dinner: Chickpea Stew

Day 6

Breakfast: Vegan Breakfast Toast

Lunch: slow-cooked Chicken and Chickpea Soup

Dinner: Garlic-Roasted Salmon with Brussels Sprouts

Day 7

Breakfast: Vegan Breakfast Toast

Lunch: slow-cooked Chicken and Chickpea Soup

Dinner: Mediterranean Cod

Week 5: Your success is within yourself

Day 1: Prep Day

Breakfast: Greek Yogurt Parfait: *Put them together one or two nights ahead for delicious, easy-grab and go meals. Consider mixing up fruit toppings for variety.*

Lunch: Vegetarian Shakshouka

Dinner: Slow Cooker Vegetarian Mediterranean Stew: *Double the recipe and use this for lunch for the week.*

Day 2

Breakfast: Greek Yogurt Parfait

Lunch: Slow Cooker Vegetarian Mediterranean Stew

Dinner: Vegan Mediterranean Buddha Bowl

Day 3

Breakfast: Greek Yogurt Parfait

Lunch: Slow Cooker Vegetarian Mediterranean Stew

Dinner: slow-cooked Brisket

Day 4

Breakfast: Greek Yogurt Parfait

Lunch: Slow Cooker Vegetarian Mediterranean Stew

Dinner: Sheet Pan Shrimp

Day 5

Breakfast: Greek Yogurt Parfait

Lunch: Slow Cooker Vegetarian Mediterranean Stew

Dinner: Herbed Lamb and Veggies

Day 6

Breakfast: Greek Yogurt Parfait

Lunch: Slow Cooker Vegetarian Mediterranean Stew

Dinner: Chicken and Couscous Mediterranean Wraps

Day 7

Breakfast: Mediterranean Breakfast Bake

Lunch: Harissa Pasta

Dinner: Vegetarian Aglio e Olio and Broccoli

Week 6: Strength is borne of struggles

Day 1: Prep Day

Breakfast: Savory Mediterranean Breakfast Muffins: Make-Ahead *for the week. You can change fillings to your taste if you'd like to change up the flavors for variety.*

Lunch: Vegetarian Greek Stuffed Mushrooms

Dinner: Slow Cooker Chicken and Chickpea Soup: *Double the batch and use for the week for lunches for the work week.*

Day 2

Breakfast: Savory Mediterranean Breakfast Muffins

Lunch: Slow Cooker Chicken and Chickpea Soup

Dinner: Vegetarian Zucchini Lasagna Rolls

Day 3

Breakfast: Savory Mediterranean Breakfast Muffins

Lunch: Slow Cooker Chicken and Chickpea Soup

Dinner: slow-cooked Brisket

Day 4

Breakfast: Savory Mediterranean Breakfast Muffins

Lunch: Slow Cooker Chicken and Chickpea Soup

Dinner: 1 Hour Baked Cod

Day 5

Breakfast: Savory Mediterranean Breakfast Muffins

Lunch: Slow Cooker Chicken and Chickpea Soup

Dinner: Herbed Lamb and Veggies

Day 6

Breakfast: Savory Mediterranean Breakfast Muffins

Lunch: Slow Cooker Chicken and Chickpea Soup

Dinner: Mediterranean Mahi Mahi

Day 7

Breakfast: Vegetarian Breakfast Sandwich

Lunch: Vegetarian Toss Together Mediterranean Salad

Dinner: Vegetarian Mediterranean Quiche

Week 7: Your only limits are your thoughts

Day 1: Prep Day

Breakfast: Mediterranean Pastry Pinwheels: *Prep ahead for the week and freeze uncooked portions to warm up while you get ready for the day.*

Lunch: Mediterranean Feta Mac and Cheese

Dinner: Spaghetti and Clams: *Save leftovers to eat for the next 2-3 days for lunch.*

Day 2

Breakfast: Mediterranean Pastry Pinwheels

Lunch: Spaghetti and Clams

Dinner: Vegan Bean Soup with Spinach

Day 3

Breakfast: Mediterranean Pastry Pinwheels

Lunch: Spaghetti and Clams

Dinner: Cilantro and Garlic Baked Salmon

Day 4

Breakfast: Mediterranean Pastry Pinwheels

Lunch: Spaghetti and Clams

Dinner: Moroccan Lentil Soup: *Prepare extra and use for lunch for the remainder of the week.*

Day 5

Breakfast: Mediterranean Pastry Pinwheels

Lunch: Moroccan Lentil Soup

Dinner: Walnut Crusted Salmon with Rosemary

Snack: Vegetarian Toss Together Mediterranean Salmon

Day 6

Breakfast: Mediterranean Pastry Pinwheels

Lunch: Moroccan Lentil Soup

Dinner: Herbed Lamb and Veggies

Day 7

Breakfast: Mediterranean Breakfast Bake

Lunch: Moroccan Lentil Soup

Dinner: Cilantro and Garlic Baked Salmon

Week 8: Stop worrying about what may go wrong and start focusing on what can go right

Day 1: Prep Day

Breakfast: Make-Ahead Overnight Oats: *Prepare a jar every night for easy breakfast for the week.*

Lunch: Grilled Chicken Mediterranean Salad

Dinner: slow-cooked Chicken and Chickpea Soup: *Double the recipe and use for work lunches for the week.*

Day 2

Breakfast: Make-Ahead Overnight Oats

Lunch: slow-cooked Chicken and Chickpea Soup

Dinner: Vegetarian Cheesy Artichoke and Spinach Stuffed Squash

Day 3

Breakfast: Make-Ahead Overnight Oats

Lunch: slow-cooked Chicken and Chickpea Soup

Dinner: Mediterranean Feta Mac and Cheese

Day 4

Breakfast: Make-Ahead Overnight Oats

Lunch: slow-cooked Chicken and Chickpea Soup

Dinner: Braised Lamb and Fennel

Day 5

Breakfast: Make-Ahead Overnight Oats

Lunch: slow-cooked Chicken and Chickpea Soup

Dinner: Baked Feta with Olive Tapenade

Day 6

Breakfast: Make-Ahead Overnight Oats

Lunch: slow-cooked Chicken and Chickpea Soup

Dinner: Vegetarian Aglio e Olio and Broccoli

Day 7

Breakfast: Vegetarian Breakfast Sandwich

Lunch: Vegetarian Greek Stuffed Mushrooms

Dinner: Vegetarian Zucchini Lasagna Rolls

Chapter 4: 12 Week Meal Plan

Week 1: The hardest part of any journey is the first step

Day 1: Prep Day

Breakfast: Savory Mediterranean Breakfast Muffins *Reserve extras for week's breakfasts*

Lunch: Aglio e Olio and Broccoli

Dinner: Slow Cooker Vegetarian Mediterranean Stew *Double recipe and reserve extras for week's lunches*

Day 2

Breakfast: Savory Mediterranean Breakfast Muffins

Lunch: Slow Cooker Vegetarian Mediterranean Stew

Dinner: Vegetarian Toss Together Mediterranean Pasta Salad

Day 3

Breakfast: Savory Mediterranean Breakfast Muffins

Lunch: Slow Cooker Vegetarian Mediterranean Stew

Dinner: Cilantro and Garlic Baked Salmon

Day 4

Breakfast: Savory Mediterranean Breakfast Muffins

Lunch: Slow Cooker Vegetarian Mediterranean Stew

Dinner: Mediterranean Mahi Mahi

Day 5

Breakfast: Savory Mediterranean Breakfast Muffins

Lunch: Slow Cooker Vegetarian Mediterranean Stew

Dinner: Grilled Chicken Mediterranean Salad

Day 6

Breakfast: Greek Yogurt Parfait

Lunch: Harissa Pasta

Dinner: Spaghetti and Clams

Day 7

Breakfast: Apple Whipped Yogurt

Lunch: Leftover Spaghetti and Clams

Dinner: Lemon Herb Chicken and Potatoes One Pot meal

Week 2: Impossible is just a big word people use when they're too afraid to change their current situation

Day 1: Prep Day

Breakfast: Make-Ahead Overnight Oats: *Set up a new jar every night before bed to have breakfast ready the next day. Change up toppings/fruits if you want some variety.*

Lunch: Chicken and Couscous Mediterranean Wraps

Dinner: Slow Cooker Chicken and Chickpea Soup: *Double the batch and take to work for the week for lunches*

Day 2

Breakfast: Make-Ahead Overnight Oats

Lunch: Slow Cooker Chicken and Chickpea Soup

Dinner: Vegetarian Greek Stuffed Mushrooms

Day 3

Breakfast: Make-Ahead Overnight Oats

Lunch: Slow Cooker Chicken and Chickpea Soup

Dinner: Sheet Pan Shrimp

Day 4

Breakfast: Make-Ahead Overnight Oats

Lunch: Slow Cooker Chicken and Chickpea Soup

Dinner: Slow Cooker Brisket: *Prepare this before work and set to low heat.*

Day 5

Breakfast: Make-Ahead Overnight Oats

Lunch: Slow Cooker Chicken and Chickpea Soup

Dinner: Grilled Chicken Mediterranean Salad

Day 6

Breakfast: Make-Ahead Overnight Oats

Lunch: Slow Cooker Chicken and Chickpea Soup

Dinner: Slow Cooker Mediterranean Chicken

Day 7

Breakfast: Make-Ahead Overnight Oats

Lunch: Mediterranean Feta Mac and Cheese

Dinner: Herbed Lamb and Veggies

Week 3: Success is failing, but getting up to try again anyway

Day 1: Prep Day

Breakfast: Mediterranean Pastry Pinwheels: *These can be frozen before they are baked and then baked individually for 10-15 minutes in a toaster oven for an easy weekday breakfast. Prepare on Sunday and reserve some for on-the-go breakfasts for the week.*

Lunch: Vegetarian Mediterranean Quiche

Dinner: Moroccan Lentil Soup: *Double this recipe and use extras for lunch for the week.*

Day 2

Breakfast: Mediterranean Pastry Pinwheels

Lunch: Moroccan Lentil Soup

Dinner: Vegetarian Zucchini Lasagna Rolls

Day 3

Breakfast: Mediterranean Pastry Pinwheels

Lunch: Moroccan Lentil Soup

Dinner: Vegan Mediterranean Buddha Bowl

Day 4

Breakfast: Mediterranean Pastry Pinwheels

Lunch: Moroccan Lentil Soup

Dinner: Lemon Herb Chicken and Potatoes One Pot Meal

Day 5

Breakfast: Mediterranean Pastry Pinwheels

Lunch: Moroccan Lentil Soup

Dinner: Chicken and Couscous Mediterranean Wrap

Day 6

Breakfast: Mediterranean Pastry Pinwheels

Lunch: Moroccan Lentil Soup

Dinner: Cilantro and Garlic Baked Salmon

Day 7

Breakfast: Mediterranean Pastry Pinwheels

Lunch: Vegan Mediterranean Pasta

Dinner: Walnut Crusted Salmon with Rosemary

Week 4: My only competition is the me from yesterday

Day 1: Prep Day

Breakfast: Vegetarian Breakfast Sandwich

Lunch: Baked Feta with Olive Tapenade

Dinner: Vegetarian Slow Cooker Quinoa: *Double and use for lunches for the week.*

Day 2

Breakfast: Vegan Breakfast Toast

Lunch: Vegetarian Slow Cooker Quinoa

Dinner: Vegetarian Cheesy Artichoke and Spinach Stuffed Squash

Day 3

Breakfast: Vegan Breakfast Toast

Lunch: Vegetarian Slow Cooker Quinoa

Dinner: Herbed Lamb and Veggies

Day 4

Breakfast: Vegetarian Breakfast Sandwich

Lunch: Vegetarian Slow Cooker Quinoa

Dinner: slow-cooked Chicken and Chickpea Soup: *Double recipe and use for lunches for the rest of the week.*

Day 5

Breakfast: Vegetarian Breakfast Sandwich

Lunch: slow-cooked Chicken and Chickpea Soup

Dinner: Chickpea Stew

Day 6

Breakfast: Vegan Breakfast Toast

Lunch: slow-cooked Chicken and Chickpea Soup

Dinner: Garlic-Roasted Salmon with Brussels Sprouts

Day 7

Breakfast: Vegan Breakfast Toast

Lunch: slow-cooked Chicken and Chickpea Soup

Dinner: Mediterranean Cod

Week 5: I can do it, and I will do it.

Day 1: Prep Day

Breakfast: Greek Yogurt Parfait: *Put them together one or two nights ahead for delicious, easy-grab and go meals. Consider mixing up fruit toppings for variety.*

Lunch: Vegetarian Shakshouka

Dinner: Slow Cooker Vegetarian Mediterranean Stew: *Double the recipe and use this for lunch for the week.*

Day 2

Breakfast: Greek Yogurt Parfait

Lunch: Slow Cooker Vegetarian Mediterranean Stew

Dinner: Vegan Mediterranean Buddha Bowl

Day 3

Breakfast: Greek Yogurt Parfait

Lunch: Slow Cooker Vegetarian Mediterranean Stew

Dinner: slow-cooked Brisket

Day 4

Breakfast: Greek Yogurt Parfait

Lunch: Slow Cooker Vegetarian Mediterranean Stew

Dinner: Sheet Pan Shrimp

Day 5

Breakfast: Greek Yogurt Parfait

Lunch: Slow Cooker Vegetarian Mediterranean Stew

Dinner: Herbed Lamb and Veggies

Day 6

Breakfast: Greek Yogurt Parfait

Lunch: Slow Cooker Vegetarian Mediterranean Stew

Dinner: Chicken and Couscous Mediterranean Wraps

Day 7

Breakfast: Mediterranean Breakfast Bake

Lunch: Harissa Pasta

Dinner: Vegetarian Aglio e Olio and Broccoli

Week 6: Success is what you make of it

Day 1: Prep Day

Breakfast: Savory Mediterranean Breakfast Muffins: Make-Ahead *for the week. You can change fillings to your taste if you'd like to change up the flavors for variety.*

Lunch: Vegetarian Greek Stuffed Mushrooms

Dinner: Slow Cooker Chicken and Chickpea Soup: *Double the batch and use for lunches for the workweek.*

Day 2

Breakfast: Savory Mediterranean Breakfast Muffins

Lunch: Slow Cooker Chicken and Chickpea Soup

Dinner: Vegetarian Zucchini Lasagna Rolls

Day 3

Breakfast: Savory Mediterranean Breakfast Muffins

Lunch: Slow Cooker Chicken and Chickpea Soup

Dinner: slow-cooked Brisket

Day 4

Breakfast: Savory Mediterranean Breakfast Muffins

Lunch: Slow Cooker Chicken and Chickpea Soup

Dinner: 1 Hour Baked Cod

Day 5

Breakfast: Savory Mediterranean Breakfast Muffins

Lunch: Slow Cooker Chicken and Chickpea Soup

Dinner: Herbed Lamb and Veggies

Day 6

Breakfast: Savory Mediterranean Breakfast Muffins

Lunch: Slow Cooker Chicken and Chickpea Soup

Dinner: Mediterranean Mahi Mahi

Day 7

Breakfast: Vegetarian Breakfast Sandwich

Lunch: Vegetarian Toss Together Mediterranean Salad

Dinner: Vegetarian Mediterranean Quiche

Week 7: Success is how high you bounce back after hitting rock bottom

Day 1: Prep Day

Breakfast: Mediterranean Pastry Pinwheels: *Prep ahead for the week and freeze uncooked portions to warm up while you get ready for the day.*

Lunch: Mediterranean Feta Mac and Cheese

Dinner: Spaghetti and Clams: *Save leftovers to eat for the next 2-3 days for lunch.*

Day 2

Breakfast: Mediterranean Pastry Pinwheels

Lunch: Spaghetti and Clams

Dinner: Vegan Bean Soup with Spinach

Day 3

Breakfast: Mediterranean Pastry Pinwheels

Lunch: Spaghetti and Clams

Dinner: Cilantro and Garlic Baked Salmon

Day 4

Breakfast: Mediterranean Pastry Pinwheels

Lunch: Spaghetti and Clams

Dinner: Moroccan Lentil Soup: *Prepare extra and use for lunch for the remainder of the week.*

Day 5

Breakfast: Mediterranean Pastry Pinwheels

Lunch: Moroccan Lentil Soup

Dinner: Walnut Crusted Salmon with Rosemary

Snack: Vegetarian Toss Together Mediterranean Salmon

Day 6

Breakfast: Mediterranean Pastry Pinwheels

Lunch: Moroccan Lentil Soup

Dinner: Herbed Lamb and Veggies

Day 7

Breakfast: Mediterranean Breakfast Bake

Lunch: Moroccan Lentil Soup

Dinner: Cilantro and Garlic Baked Salmon

Week 8: Success is defined by your own terms

Day 1: Prep Day

Breakfast: Make-Ahead Overnight Oats: *Prepare a jar every night for easy breakfast for the week.*

Lunch: Grilled Chicken Mediterranean Salad

Dinner: slow-cooked Chicken and Chickpea Soup: *Double the recipe and use for work lunches for the week.*

Day 2

Breakfast: Make-Ahead Overnight Oats

Lunch: slow-cooked Chicken and Chickpea Soup

Dinner: Vegetarian Cheesy Artichoke and Spinach Stuffed Squash

Day 3

Breakfast: Make-Ahead Overnight Oats

Lunch: slow-cooked Chicken and Chickpea Soup

Dinner: Mediterranean Feta Mac and Cheese

Day 4

Breakfast: Make-Ahead Overnight Oats

Lunch: slow-cooked Chicken and Chickpea Soup

Dinner: Braised Lamb and Fennel

Day 5

Breakfast: Make-Ahead Overnight Oats

Lunch: slow-cooked Chicken and Chickpea Soup

Dinner: Baked Feta with Olive Tapenade

Day 6

Breakfast: Make-Ahead Overnight Oats

Lunch: slow-cooked Chicken and Chickpea Soup

Dinner: Vegetarian Aglio e Olio and Broccoli

Day 7

Breakfast: Vegetarian Breakfast Sandwich

Lunch: Vegetarian Greek Stuffed Mushrooms

Dinner: Vegetarian Zucchini Lasagna Rolls

Week 9: Happiness is the key to succeeding

Day 1: Prep Day

Breakfast: Savory Mediterranean Breakfast Muffins: *Make extras and enjoy them all week long.*

Lunch: Vegetarian Toss Together Mediterranean Pasta Salad: *Make extras and enjoy this cold all week for lunch.*

Dinner: Mediterranean Cod

Day 2

Breakfast: Savory Mediterranean Breakfast Muffins

Lunch: Vegetarian Toss Together Mediterranean Pasta Salad

Dinner: Harissa Pasta

Day 3

Breakfast: Savory Mediterranean Breakfast Muffins

Lunch: Vegetarian Toss Together Mediterranean Pasta Salad

Dinner: Garlic-Roasted Salmon and Brussels Sprouts

Day 4

Breakfast: Savory Mediterranean Breakfast Muffins

Lunch: Vegetarian Toss Together Mediterranean Pasta Salad

Dinner: Vegetarian Aglio e Olio and Broccoli

Day 5

Breakfast: Savory Mediterranean Breakfast Muffins

Lunch: Vegetarian Toss Together Mediterranean Pasta Salad

Dinner: Lemon Herb Chicken and Potatoes One Pot Meal

Day 6

Breakfast: Savory Mediterranean Breakfast Muffins

Lunch: Vegetarian Toss Together Mediterranean Pasta Salad

Dinner: Cilantro and Garlic Baked Salmon

Day 7

Breakfast: Vegan Breakfast Toast

Lunch: Vegan Mediterranean Buddha Bowl

Dinner: Slow Cooker Mediterranean Chicken

Week 10: Work every day for the success you desire

Day 1: Prep Day

Breakfast: Vegetarian Breakfast Sandwich*: Buy extra ingredients and quickly fry up an egg each morning for a healthy, hearty breakfast.*

Lunch: Grilled Chicken Mediterranean Salad

Dinner: Moroccan Lentil Soup: *Make extra and enjoy this all week long for lunch*

Day 2

Breakfast: Vegetarian Breakfast Sandwich

Lunch: Moroccan Lentil Soup

Dinner: Vegetarian Greek Stuffed Mushrooms

Day 3

Breakfast: Vegetarian Breakfast Sandwich

Lunch: Moroccan Lentil Soup

Dinner: slow-cooked Brisket

Day 4

Breakfast: Vegetarian Breakfast Sandwich

Lunch: Moroccan Lentil Soup

Dinner: Slow Cooker Mediterranean Chicken

Day 5

Breakfast: Vegetarian Breakfast Sandwich

Lunch: Moroccan Lentil Soup

Dinner: Cilantro and Garlic Baked Salmon

Day 6

Breakfast: Vegetarian Breakfast Sandwich

Lunch: Moroccan Lentil Soup

Dinner: 1 Hour Baked Cod

Day 7

Breakfast: Mediterranean Breakfast Bake

Lunch: Chicken and Couscous Mediterranean Wraps

Dinner: Mediterranean Mahi Mahi

Week 11: Success is nothing but perseverance and learning from failure

Day 1: Prep Day

Breakfast: Make-Ahead Overnight Oats: *Prepare these every night for easy grab and go breakfasts*

Lunch: Sheet Pan Shrimp

Dinner: Spaghetti and Clams: *Reserve leftovers for the next few days for lunches.*

Day 2

Breakfast: Make-Ahead Overnight Oats

Lunch: Spaghetti and Clams

Dinner: Vegetarian Mediterranean Pasta

Day 3

Breakfast: Make-Ahead Overnight Oats

Lunch: Spaghetti and Clams

Dinner: Slow-Cooked Brisket

Day 4

Breakfast: Make-Ahead Overnight Oats

Lunch: Spaghetti and Clams

Dinner: Moroccan Lentil Soup: *Reserve leftovers for the next few days of lunches.*

Day 5

Breakfast: Make-Ahead Overnight Oats

Lunch: Moroccan Lentil Soup

Dinner: Slow Cooker Mediterranean Chicken

Snack:

Day 6

Breakfast: Make-Ahead Overnight Oats

Lunch: Moroccan Lentil Soup

Dinner: Vegetarian Zucchini Lasagna Rolls

Day 7

Breakfast: Vegan Breakfast Toast

Lunch: Mediterranean Feta Mac and Cheese

Dinner: Chickpea Stew

Week 12: Success is earned one step at a time, one day at a time, one minute at a time

Day 1: Prep Day

Breakfast: Mediterranean Pastry Pinwheels: *Prepare extra and keep them stored in freezer unbaked, baking one or two slices for breakfast on the go.*

Lunch: Baked Feta with Olive Tapenade

Dinner: Slow Cooker Vegetarian Mediterranean Stew: *Double recipe and use all week for lunches.*

Day 2

Breakfast: Mediterranean Pastry Pinwheels

Lunch: Slow Cooker Vegetarian Mediterranean Stew

Dinner: Vegan Mediterranean Buddha Bowl

Day 3

Breakfast: Mediterranean Pastry Pinwheels

Lunch: Slow Cooker Vegetarian Mediterranean Stew

Dinner: 1 Hour Baked Cod

Day 4

Breakfast: Mediterranean Pastry Pinwheels

Lunch: Slow Cooker Vegetarian Mediterranean Stew

Dinner:

Day 5

Breakfast: Mediterranean Pastry Pinwheels

Lunch: Slow Cooker Vegetarian Mediterranean Stew

Dinner: Sheet Pan Shrimp

Day 6

Breakfast: Mediterranean Pastry Pinwheels

Lunch: Slow Cooker Vegetarian Mediterranean Stew

Dinner: Walnut Crusted Salmon with Rosemary

Day 7

Breakfast: Vegetarian Breakfast Sandwich

Lunch: Vegetarian Aglio e Olio and Broccoli

Dinner: Cilantro and Garlic Baked Salmon

Chapter 5: Maintaining Your Diet

Sticking to a diet can be tough. You could see that other people are having some great food and wish that you could enjoy it too. You might realize that you miss the foods that you used to eat and feel like it's a drag to not be able to enjoy them. When you are able to enjoy the foods that you are eating, sticking to your diet is far easier. However, that doesn't mean that you won't miss those old foods sometimes. Thankfully, the Mediterranean diet is not a very restrictive one—you are able to enjoy foods in moderation that would otherwise not be allowed, and because of that, you can take the slice of cake at the work party, or you can choose to pick up a coffee for yourself every now and then. When you do this, you're not doing anything wrong, so long as you enjoy food in moderation.

Within this chapter, we are going to take a look at several tips that you can use that will help you with maintaining your diet so that you will be able to stick to it, even when you feel like things are getting difficult. Think of this as your guide to avoiding giving in entirely—this will help you to do the best thing for yourself so that you can know that you are healthy. Now, let's get started.

Find Your Motivation

First, if you want to keep yourself on your diet, one of the best things that you can do is make sure that you find and stick to your motivation. Make sure that you know what it is in life that is motivating you. Are you losing weight because a doctor told you to? Fair enough—but how do you make that personal and about yourself? Maybe instead of looking at it as a purely health-related choice, look at it as something that you are doing because of yourself. Maybe you are eating better so that you are able to watch your children graduate or so that you can run after them at the park and stay healthy, even when it is hard to do so.

Remind Yourself Why You are Eating Healthily

When you find that you are struggling to eat healthily, remind yourself of why you are doing it in the first place. When you do this enough, you will begin to resist the urges easier than ever. Make it a point to tell yourself not to eat something a certain way. Take the time to remind yourself that you don't need to order that greasy pizza—you are eating better foods because you want to be there for your children or grandchildren.

Reminding yourself of your motivation is a great way to overcome those cravings that you may have at any point in time. The cravings that you have are usually strong and compelling, but if you learn to overcome them, you realize that they weren't actually as powerful as you thought they were. Defeat the cravings. Learn to tell yourself that they are not actually able to control you. Tell yourself that you can do better with yourself.

Eat Slowly

Now, on the Mediterranean diet, you should already be eating your meals with other people anyway. You should be taking the time to enjoy those meals while talking to other people and ensuring that you get that connection with them, and in doing so, you realize that you are able to do better. You realize that you are able to keep yourself under control longer, and that is a great way to defend and protect yourself from overeating.

When you eat slowly, you can get the same effect. Eating slowly means that you will have longer for your brain to realize that you should be eating less. When you are able to trigger that sensation of satiety because you were eating slowly, you end up eating fewer calories by default, and that matters immensely.

Keep Yourself Accountable

Don't forget that, ultimately, your diet is something that you must control on your own. Keep yourself accountable by making sure that you show other people what you are doing. If you are trying to lose weight, let them know, and tell them how you plan to do so. When you do this, you are able to remind yourself that other people know what you are doing and why—this is a great way to foster that sense of accountability because you will feel like you have to actually follow through, or you will be embarrassed by having to admit fault. You could also make accountability to yourself as well. When you do this, you are able to remind yourself that your diet is your own. Using apps to track your food and caloric intake is just one way that you can do this.

Remember Your Moderation

While it can be difficult to face a diet where you feel like you can't actually enjoy the foods that you would like to eat, the truth is that on the Mediterranean diet, you are totally okay to eat those foods that you like or miss if you do so in moderation. There is nothing that is absolutely forbidden on the Mediterranean diet—there are just foods that you should be restricting regularly. However, that doesn't mean that you can't have a treat every now and then.

Remembering to live in moderation will help you from feeling like you have to cheat or give up as well. When you are able to enjoy your diet and still enjoy the times where you want to enjoy your treats, you realize that there is actually a happy medium between sticking to the diet and deciding to quit entirely.

Identify the Difference between Hunger and Craving

Another great way to help yourself stick to your diet is to recognize that there is a very real difference between actually being hungry and just craving something to eat. In general, cravings are felt in the mouth—when you feel like you are salivating or like you need to eat something, but it is entirely in your head and mouth, you know that you have a craving. When you are truly hungry, you feel an emptiness in your stomach—you are able to know because your abdomen is where the motivation is coming from.

Being able to tell when you have a craving and when you are genuinely hungry, you can usually avoid eating extra calories that you didn't actually need. This is major—if you don't want to overeat, you need to know when your body actually needs something and when it just wants something. And if you find that you just want something, that's okay too—just find a way to move on from it. If you want to indulge a bit here and there, there's no harm in that!

Stick to the Meal Plan

When it comes to sticking to a diet, one of the easiest and most straightforward ways to do so is to just stick to your meal plan that you set up. You have it there for a reason—it is there for you to fall back on, and the sooner that you are willing to accept that, recognizing that ultimately, you can stay on track when you don't have to think about things too much, the better you will do. You will be able to succeed on your diet because you will know that you have those tools in place to protect you—they will be lined up to ensure that your diet is able to provide you with everything that you need and they will also be there so that you can know that you are on the right track.

Drink Plenty of Water

Another key to keeping yourself on track with your diet is to make sure that you drink plenty of water throughout the day. Oftentimes, we mistake our thirst with hunger and eat instead. Of course, if you're thirsty, food isn't going to really fix your problem, and you will end up continuing to mix up the sensation as you try to move past it. The more you eat, the thirstier you will get until you realize that you're full but still feeling "hungry." By drinking plenty of water any time that you think that you might want to eat, you will be able to keep yourself hydrated, and in addition, you will prevent yourself from unintentionally eating too much.

Eat Several Times Per Day

One of the best ways to keep yourself on track with your diet is to make sure that you are regularly eating. By eating throughout the day, making sure that you keep yourself full, it is easier to keep yourself strong enough to resist giving in to cravings or anything else. When you do this regularly, you will discover that you can actually keep away much of your cravings so that you are more successful in managing your diet.

Eating several times per day often involves small meals and snacks if you prefer to do so. Some people don't like doing this, but if you find that you're one of those people who will do well on a diet when you are never actually hungry enough to get desperate enough to break it, you will probably be just fine.

Fill Up on Protein

Another great way to protect yourself from giving in and caving on your diet is to make sure that you fill up on protein. Whether it comes from an animal or plant source, make sure that every time you eat, you have some sort of tangible protein source. This is the best way to keep yourself on track because protein keeps you fuller for longer. When you eat something that's loaded up with protein, you don't feel the need to eat as much later on. The protein is usually very dense, and that means that you get to resist feeling hungry for longer than you thought that you would.

Some easy proteins come from nuts—but make sure that you are mindful that you do not end up overeating during this process—you might unintentionally end up eating too many without realizing it. While you should be eating proteins regularly, make sure that you are mindful of calorie content as well!

Keep Only Healthy Foods

A common mistake that people make while dieting is that they end up caving when they realize that their home is filled up with foods that they shouldn't be eating. Perhaps you are the only person in your home that is attempting to diet. In this case, you may end up running into a situation where you have all sorts of non-compliant foods on hand. You might have chips for your kids or snacks that your partner likes to eat on hand. You may feel like it is difficult for you to stay firm when you have that to consider, and that means that you end up stuck in temptation.

One of the best ways to prevent this is to either cut all of the unhealthy junk out of your home entirely or make sure that you keep the off-limits foods in specific places so that you don't have to look at it and see it tempting you every time that you go to get a snack for yourself. By trying to keep yourself limited to just healthy foods, you will be healthier, and you will make better decisions.

Eat Breakfast Daily

Finally, make sure that breakfast is non-negotiable. Make sure that you enjoy it every single day, even if you're busy. This is where those make-ahead meals can come in handy; by knowing that you have to keep to a meal plan and knowing that you already have the food on hand, you can keep yourself fed. Breakfast sets you up for success or failure—if you want to truly succeed on your diet, you must make sure that you are willing to eat those healthier foods as much as possible, and you must get started on the right foot. Enjoy those foods first thing every day. Eat so that you are not ravenous when you finally do decide that it is time to sit down and find something to eat. Even if you just have a smoothie or something quick to eat as you go, having breakfast will help you to persevere.

PART III

Chapter 1: The Power of the Crock Pot and Its Benefits

The Ways You Can Benefit

Think of how many times you have experienced 'spells' that you did not feel like spending hours over the stove preparing dinner. Can you relate? How about the times during the holidays when you are planning on a houseful of guests; yikes? By the way, "Don't sweat it because you have your fabulous cooker and all of these new recipes to try out."

These are a few ways to make the path a bit easier:

Get Ahead of the Meal: Preparing food with your Crock-Pot® can put you ahead of the game the night before you have a busy day planned. You can always make the meal for the next day in just a few minutes. Put all of the ingredients (if they can combine overnight) into the pot, so when you get up the next morning; all you need to do is take it out of the fridge, and let it get to room temperature. Turn it on as you head out of the door and dinner will be ready when you get home. YES!

Save a lot of Effort and Time: All it takes is a few good recipes and a little bit of your valuable time. In most of the cases, these recipes are geared towards a fast lifestyle and will be ready with just a few simple steps. After some time and practice, you will know exactly which ones will be your favorites; all of them!

Cut Back on Dining Out: Having an enjoyable meal at home is so much more personal for your family because you (and your pot) prepared it! Not only that, You will eliminate the temptation to order foods that might not be so healthy and in turn—will be more expensive.

Watching the Extra Liquids: There is no need to use additional ingredients, other than what is described within each of the recipes. Ideally, you should not fill the more than half to two-thirds full of ingredients. Too much liquid will cause a leakage from the top and may result in improperly cooked food.

Cook it Slow & Leave it Alone: A slow cooker is known for creating delicious dishes while bringing out all of the natural flavors. So, go ahead and go to work or have some fun—or—better yet go to bed early! There is no need to worry about checking on it (unless the recipe calls for it). Each time the lid is removed—valuable heat is escaping—resulting in a breakdown of the advised times. Just keep that element it in mind, even though it smells so good!

Trimming the Fat: One huge advantage to the use of this type of cooking is you can save quite a chunk of money purchasing cheaper cuts of meat. Also, capitalize on the flavorful meat in small quantities and by bulking up on veggies with smaller meat portions.

Hot Antioxidants

Many recent studies have discovered cooking some food items such as tomatoes will increase the bioavailability of many of the nutrients. For example, lycopene which is linked to cancer and heart prevention becomes move available to the body because the heat releases the lycopene.

A study from 2003 compared the content of fresh, frozen, and canned corn which was processed with heat; specifically lutein and xeaxanthin, and found less lutein in the fresh version. This lutein is mostly well-known to protect you from some eye diseases.

Score 'ONE' for the Crock-Pot®.

Who Knew?

Basic Times & Settings

The question always arises of how long you should cook your items if you don't have a recipe for a Crock-Pot®. These are only general guidelines because the size of a pot will make a difference in the cooking times.

Regular Cooking	Crock Pot® High Temperatures	Crock Pot® Low Pot Temperatures

Times

Hours

1/4 to 1/2	1 to 2	4 to 6
1/2 to 1	2 to 3	5 to 7
1 to 2	3 to 4	6 to 8
2 to 4	4 to 6	8 to 12

Note: You must consider that root veggies take longer than other vegetables and meats which mean they should be placed in the lower part of the pot.

Are You Ready? Of course, you are!

Chapter 2: Healthy Breakfast Recipes

Boiled Eggs

Did you ever wake up in the middle of the night for a 'potty' break, and decided you want some boiled eggs or egg salad for breakfast or work tomorrow, but do not have the time to sit around and wait for the eggs to cook? You have a cure for that!

Ingredients and Instructions

The simplicity is amazing!

1) Pour some water into the Crock-Pot®, add as many eggs as you want, and set the pot for 3 ½ hours on the low setting. Go back to bed and enjoy tomorrow!

One-Hour Bread

Crave that fresh bread—no longer! You can have some delicious comfort food shortly!

Ingredients

1 ½ C. Baking Mix

3 Tbsp. Italian Seasoning

½ cup milk (skim is okay)

Optional: ½ C. shredded cheese or 3 Tbsp. Grated Parmesan cheese

Directions

1) Prepare the cooker with some non-stick cooking spray.

2) Combine all of the ingredients until the lumps are gone and empty into the cooker.

3) *Notes:* Bisquick® is a good choice.

Breakfast Fiesta Delight

Directions
1 Pound Country-Style Sausage
1 Package (28-ounces) frozen hash brown potatoes (thawed)
½ Cup whole milk
12 large eggs
1 ½ Cups shredded Mexican blend cheese
Directions

1) Prepare the Crock-Pot® by spraying it with some cooking spray to help with the cleanup.

2) Brown and crumble the sausage in a frying pan; remove and pat the grease away using a paper towel.

3) Whip the eggs together in a mixing container.

4) Layer the ingredients with a layer of potatoes, cheese, sausage, and eggs.

5) *Serving Time*: Have some salsa, sour cream, pepper, and salt for a tasty topping.

Servings: Six to Eight
Prep Time is fifteen minutes
Cooking Time is six to eight hours.
Italian Sausage Scramble
Ingredients
1 ½ Lbs. Italian sausage
1 medium yellow onion
6 medium red potatoes
¼ Cup fresh Italian minced parsley
One medium diced tomato
1 Cup frozen/fresh kernel corn
2 cups grated Cheddar cheese
Directions
1) Discard the outer casing from the sausage. Peel and dice the onions and potatoes.

2) Sauté the onion and crumbled sausage until browned. Place them on a few paper towels to absorb the grease/fat and add the items to the slow cooker.

3) Combine the rest of the ingredients—blending well. Cover and cook.

Servings: Six
Prep Time is 15 Minutes.
Cook Time: The high setting is for four hours, and the lower setting is for six to eight hours.

The Sweeter Side of Breakfast
Blueberry Steel Cut Oats
Ingredients
1 ½ C. of water
2 C. frozen blueberries
1 banana
1 C. Steel cut oats
1- ½ C. Vanilla almond milk
1 Tbsp. butter
1 ½ tsp. cinnamon
Directions
1) Prepare a six-quart cooker with the butter, making sure to cover the sides also.

2) Mash the banana slightly and add all of the ingredients into the Pot—stirring gently.

3) Place the top on the crock pot and cook for *one hour* on the HIGH setting; switch to the WARM setting overnight, and sleep tight!

Wake up ready for a busy day by adding a drizzle of honey and get moving!

Servings: Four to Six

Preparation Time: Fifteen Minutes

Cooking Time: Eight hours

Pumpkin Pie Oatmeal

Ingredients

1 C. oats (steel cut)

3 ½ C. water

1 C. pumpkin puree

¼ tsp. each:

- salt

- vanilla extract

- pumpkin pie spices

Optional: 2 Tbsp. maple syrup

Directions

1) Use some non-stick cooking spray to coat the Crock-Pot®.

2) Empty the oats into the Pot.

3) Mix the remainder of the ingredients in a large mixing container, and pour over the oats.

4) *Note:* If you like sweeter oatmeal just adjust the flavor after it is

cooked.

Cooking Time: Eight hours on low

Pumpkin Butter
Ingredients
4 Cups pumpkin
1 tsp. ground ginger
2 tsp. cinnamon
1-¼ Cups honey/maple syrup
½ tsp. nutmeg
1 tsp. vanilla extract (*optional*)
Instructions

1) Blend the vanilla, syrup/honey, and pumpkin puree in the Crock-

   Pot®.

2) Cover and cook. During the last hour—add the ginger,

   cinnamon, and nutmeg.

3) If you want it a little thicker, you can crack the lid. After all, the

   aroma is tantalizing—especially first thing in the morning!

You can store in jars in the bottom of the fridge for a healthy addition—
anytime.
Yields: About 10 ounces
Preparation Time: Five Minutes
Cooking Time: Five hours

Chapter 3: Time-Saving Lunch Specialties

Beef Tacos

Ingredients

1 Package taco seasoning

1 (ten-ounce) Can tomatoes and green chilies (Rotel)

1 Pound lean ground beef

Directions

1) Add everything listed into your Crock-Pot®.

2) If you are available; stir every couple of hours to break up the beef or break it up before serving.

3) Serve on a floured tortilla or taco shell with your choice of toppings.

Servings: 12 tacos

Preparation Time: Two Minutes

Cooking Time: Five to Six Hours

Root Beer & BBQ Chicken

Ingredients

1 (18-ounce) bottle barbecue sauce

4 chicken breasts

¼ teaspoon each pepper and salt

½ can or bottle root beer (full-sugar)

Note: You can use Dr. Pepper or Coke instead of root beer.

Directions

1) Pour the drink of choice, and place the chicken in the cooker.

2) Drain once the chicken has finished cooking, and discard most of the liquid—but leaving enough to prevent dryness.

3) Flavor with some pepper and salt if desired and empty the contents of the sauce into the Crock-Pot®, cooking for about 15 to 20 minutes.

4) Enjoy on some burger buns or rolls.

Cooking Time: The high temperature will have it ready in 3 hours.

Stuffed Banana Peppers

Ingredients

1 Package Italian Sausage
Banana Peppers
2 Jars of Marinara Sauce (approximately)

Directions

1) Adapt this for your crowd on the amounts used.

2) Remove both ends of the peppers and scoop out the seeds and discard them.

3) Pour ½ of the jar of sauce in the Crock-Pot®.

4) Dice the sausage, in case it is not already prepared.

5) Stuff the pepper with the sausage and put them into the Pot.

6) Pour the sauce over the banana peppers.

Cooking Time: Low for eight to nine hours

Crock-Pot® Taco Soup

Ingredients

1 (14.5-ounces) Can Each:

- Beef broth

- Petite diced tomatoes

1 (15-ounces) Can Each:

- Black beans

- Corn

1 (10-ounces) Can Rotel Original

1 Can kidney beans (16-ounces)

1 (1-oz.) pouch each:

- Taco seasoning mix

- Ranch seasoning mix (Hidden Valley)

½ teaspoon salt

1 ½ teaspoons onion powder

1 Lb. ground beef

Garnish: Sour Cream, Fritos, chopped green onions, or some shredded cheddar cheese

Notes: The recipe is excellent if you choose the 'Diced Tomatoes with Green Chilies.'

Directions

1) Cook the beef and drain. Rinse and drain all of the cans of veggies except for the chilies; reserve the liquid from the corn and tomatoes.

2) Toss everything into the Crock-Pot® (except for the garnishes).

3) Cook for the necessary time.

4) When the process is completed, add the garnishes of your choice

with some Fritos on the side to complement the flavors

Servings: 8 to 10

Prep Time: Ten minutes

Cook Time: Low for 4 hrs. or High for 2 hrs.

Chapter 4: Dinner in a Hurry
Beef
Meat for the Tacos
Ingredients

2 Lbs. Ground beef (lean)

1 cup diced onions/Birds Eye Chopped Onions and Garlic

1 Package low-sodium taco seasoning mix

Directions

1) Put the burger into the Crock-Pot® and cook it for four to six hours. If you are in the area of the kitchen—stir the meat every couple of hours to ensure it is cooking evenly (if not—no worries).

2) When the cooking cycle is complete; drain the beef on some paper towels.

3) Combine the onions and ½ to one package of the taco seasoning.

4) Blend well and continue cooking for about one more hour

Servings: Six

Preparation Time: Five Minutes

Cooking Time: Low setting: Four to Six hours

Steak Pizzaiola

Ingredients

1 (one to two pounds) London Broil

1 Yellow, orange, or red sliced bell pepper

1 Large sliced onion

¼ Cup water

½ to ¾ of a jar (your choice) tomato pasta sauce

Directions

1) Flavor the meat with the pepper and salt and place it into the Crock-Pot®.

2) Add the peppers and onions, followed by your favorite sauce,

3) Cook for six to eight hours. (Flip a time or two if you are home.)

4) Serve over some pasta, potatoes, or veggies.

Cooking Time: Low heat for six to eight hours

Steaks in the Pot

Ingredients

4 to 6 steaks

¼ C. White Wine

2 T. A-1 Sauce

2 T. Dijon mustard

Directions

1) Blend the mustard and steak sauce; add it to each of the pieces of steak.

2) Add the meat into the Crock-Pot®, add the wine, and cook for six to eight hours.

Servings: Four or More

Cooking Time: 6 to 8 Hours on the low setting

Chicken and Turkey

Buffalo Chicken

Ingredients
3 to 5 Pounds (no skin or bones) chicken breasts
1 (12-ounce) Bottle Red Hot Wings Buffalo Sauce
1 Pouch ranch dressing mix
Directions

1) Put the chicken into the Crock-Pot®. Empty the sauce over the breasts and sprinkle the ranch mix over the top. Cover and Cook.

2) Take the chicken out of the Pot and throw away the sauce.

3) Shred the chicken with a couple of forks. It should be tender.

4) Put it back into the cooker and stir to coat the chicken thoroughly.

5) Leave it in the pot on low about one more hour. Most of the sauce will be absorbed.

Cooking Time: Low for five hours

Caesar Chicken

Ingredients
1 bottle (12-ounces) Caesar dressing
4 skinless & boneless chicken breasts

½ Cup shredded Parmesan cheese

Directions

1) Add the breasts of chicken to the Crock-Pot®.

2) Cook the chicken for the specified time and drain the juices.

3) Empty the dressing over the breasts.

4) Sprinkle the cheese on top of that and cook for thirty more minutes covered until done.

Have a side of Caesar salad to complement the meal.

Servings: Four

Prep Time: 5 minutes

Cooking Time: Use the low setting for 6 hrs. ; the high setting High for 3 hrs.

Cranberry Chicken

Ingredients

4 (no skin or bones) Chicken Breasts

1 (8-ounces) bottle Kraft Catalina dressing

1 Pouch dry onion soup
1 (14-ounces) Can Ocean Spray Whole Cranberry Sauce

Directions

1) Cook the chicken in the Crock-Pot® according to your specified times. Drain the juices.

2) Combine the cranberry sauce, onion soup mix, and dressing. Empty it over the chicken.

3) Cook—covered—about 30 minutes.

Servings: Four

Preparation Time: Five minutes

Cooking Time: High for three hours or low for six hours

French Onion Chicken

Ingredients

4 Chicken breasts (no bones or skin)

1 Can French Onion soup (10.5-ounces)
½ cup sour cream

Directions

1) Put the breasts in the Pot and cook for the stated time. Empty

   the liquids.

2) Combine the soup and sour cream and add into the pot on top of

   the chicken

breasts.

3) Cook covered for about 30 minutes.

Servings: Four
Preparation Time: Five Minutes
Cooking Time: The high setting will take approximately three hours, whereas the low setting takes six hours.
Hawaiian Chicken
Ingredients

4 to 5 skinless and boneless breasts of chicken (thawed)

1 (20-oz.) Can Dole Pineapple Chunks

1 Bottle (12-oz.) Heinz Chili Sauce

1/3 C. brown sugar

Directions

1) Cook the chicken until its predetermined time limit is completed. Empty the liquid.

2) Combine the brown sugar, ½ of the juices of the can of pineapples, the chili sauce, and the chunks of pineapple.

3) Empty the mixture over the drained breasts and heat on the high setting for approximately 30 minutes or so.

4) Have a bit of pineapple in every bite. Yummy!

Servings: 4 to 5

Preparation Time: 5 min.

Cooking Time: High = 6 hrs. / Low = 3 hrs.

Honey Mustard Chicken

Ingredients
1 (12-ounces) Bottle Dijon mustard
1/3 C. honey
4 skinless & boneless chicken breasts (thawed)

Directions

1) Cook the chicken for its predetermined time and dispose of the juices.

2) Combine the mustard and honey in a small dish.

3) Empty the sauce over the chicken and cook for about ½ hour (covered) until done,

Servings: Four
Preparation Time: Five Minutes

Cooking Time: Use the low setting for six hrs. Or on high for three hrs.

Chicken Italian Style

Ingredients

4 chicken breasts (thawed – no bones- no skin)

1 (16-ounce) Bottle Italian Dressing

Directions

1) Place the breasts of chicken into your Crock-Pot® and pour the

    dressing on them.

2) Put the lid on and let it do your work!

Servings: Four

Preparation Time: 5 minutes

Cooking Time: Use the high setting to prepare the chicken for 3.5 hrs. Or use the low setting for 7 hours.

Swedish Meatballs

Ingredients

1 (12-ounce) jar Heinz HomeStyle Gravy (Savory Beef)

1 (eight-ounce) container of sour cream

1 Bag Frozen Meatballs

Instructions

1) Empty the gravy into the Crock-Pot®, followed by the sour

    cream.

2) Combine these until they are completely blended.

3) Toss the package of frozen meatballs into the Pot filling to

    approximately 2/3 to ¾ of the space.

4) Place the lid on the pot and cook—occasionally stirring if you

    happen to be close to the kitchen.

5) You can always make more or less of the recipe depending on how many people you will serve.

Cooking Time: Low for a minimum of 5 hours

Sweet and Sour Chicken

Ingredients

1 (22-ounces) Bag frozen Tyson Chicken Breast
2 Cups cooked rice/steamed vegetables (or both)
1 bottle (18-ounces) Apricot Preserves
1 jar (12-ounces) chili sauce

Directions

1) Layer the frozen chicken pieces into the Crock-Pot®.

2) Combine the preserves and chili sauce in a small container (a mixing cup is ideal). Empty it over the chicken. *Note:* You can also use pineapple or a combination.

3) Toss to mix and let the Pot do the work.

4) Enjoy with some veggies and rice.

Servings: Six (one cup per serving)
Cooking Time on the high setting is 2 to 3 hours.

Creamy Taco Chicken

Ingredients

1 Can Rotel Original Tomatoes with Green Chilies
3 chicken breasts (no bone or skin)
4-ounces cream cheese (regular or light)

Directions

1) Pour the tomatoes, and place the chicken into the slow cooker.

2) A few minutes before the end of the cooking cycle, use a fork or tongs to shred the chicken.

3) Put the cream cheese on top of the mixture, but don't stir.

4) By the time the meal is ready, the cheese will be oozing into your chicken. Yummy!

Suggestions: You can use this in a casserole, over rice, as a salad, or any other creative plan you may have for your meal.

Cooking Time: Low temperature - Six to Eight hours

Stuffed – Roasted Turkey

Ingredients

2 C. Stuffing Mix

Black pepper and salt

6 Pounds Turkey

1 Tablespoon melted butter

Instructions

1) Use the package instructions to prepare the stuffing.

2) Flavor the turkey with some melted butter, pepper, and salt.

3) Prepare the bird by loosely placing the stuffing in the carcass.

4) Cover and let the Pot do the rest.

Servings: Four

Cooking Time: Low: 9 to 11 hours; High: 5 hours

Fish

Citrus Flavored Fish

Ingredients

Pepper and Salt

1 ½ pounds fish fillets

1 medium chopped onion

4 tsp. oil

5 Tbsp. Chopped parsley

2 tsp. Each grated: lemon and orange rind

Garnish: Lemon and orange slices

Directions

Use some butter to grease the Crock-Pot®.

1) Flavor the fish with some pepper and salt and put it into the pot.

2) Add the parsley, grated rinds, and onion as well as the oil over the fish.

3) Cover and cook.

4) When ready to eat; garnish with some lemon or orange slices.

Cooking Time: 1 ½ Hours on Low

Salmon Bake

Ingredients

3 (one-pound) Cans Salmon

1 (16-ounces) can tomato puree

4 cups bread crumbs (10 slices worth)

1 chopped green pepper

3 teaspoons lemon juice

2 crushed chicken bouillon cubes

1 Can each (condensed) cream of onion soup & cream of celery soup

6 (well-beaten) eggs

½ cup milk

Directions

1) Use some cooking spray or other oil to grease the Crock-Pot® lightly.

2) Blend all of the ingredients—except for the milk and celery soup into the Pot.

3) Cover and cook.

4) Combine and stir the milk and celery soup in a small pan to use as a sauce for the salmon.

5) When the salmon is done, garnish and enjoy with the special sauce!

Cooking Time: High for three hours or low for four to six hours

Pork

BBQ Style Pork Steaks

Ingredients

4 (½-inch cut) Pork shoulder steaks

2 large sliced tomatoes

1 large onion

1 large thinly sliced bell pepper

1 Tbsp. Each:

- Vegetable oil

- Tapioca (quick-cooking)

¼ C. red wine

½ tsp. cumin

½ C. barbecue sauce (your choice)

Directions

1) Slice and cut the onion as if you are preparing to make onion rings for dinner.

2) Trim away an excess fat and slice the steaks in half - lengthwise.

3) Brown the steaks in skillet using hot oil, and drain on paper towels.

4) Organize the peppers, tomatoes, and onions in the Crock-Pot®; sprinkling the tapioca over them. Place the pork in last.

5) Prepare the cumin, wine, and barbecue sauce in a small dish. Pour it over the ingredients in the Pot, and cover.

Servings: Four
Cooking Time: Low Heat – Six to Eight Hours (or until veggies and meat are tender)
Note: The recipe is based on a 3 ½- or a 4-quart Crock-Pot®. If you have a different size the cooking time may vary.

Pepsi® Roast

Ingredients
1 Can Cream of mushroom soup
5 Lb. Pork Roast/ Steak/Chops
½ package dry onion soup mix
1 can Regular Pepsi (Don't use Diet)

Directions
1) Put the meat in the Crock-Pot® first and sprinkle with the soup mix.

2) Empty the mushroom soup and Pepsi over the meat.

3) Close the lid and let the pot do the rest of the chore.

Suggestion: Use the sauce to pour over some rice or potatoes.
Servings: Eight
Cooking Time: Low setting for six to seven hours

Ranch Chops

Ingredients
Pouch – Ranch Dressing Mix
Pork Chops

1 Can Cream of Chicken Soup Plus (+) 1 Can Water OR 2 Cups Cream of Chicken

Directions

1) Pour the liquids into the Crock-Pot® along with the chops and dressing mix.

Cooking Time: Use the low-temperature setting for four to six hours.

Ham in Cider Gravy

This ham is so tasty it cannot remain in the 'breakfast only' slot. It is so tasty and can advance to lunch and dinner menus as well.

Ingredients

1 (one to four pound) Ham
¾ cup maple syrup
2 cups unsweetened apple cider
3 Tablespoons cornstarch

Directions

1) Arrange the ham in the Crock-Pot® and top it off with the syrup and cider.

2) Cook until the time indicated below is completed.

3) Move the ham to a serving platter. Pour the liquid into a large cup (a measuring cup is perfect).

4) Whisk ½ of the cider and the cornstarch on the stovetop using the low-temperature setting until it is smooth. Continue whisking and increase the burner to med-low—adding small amounts of cider at a time—until the gravy is bubbly and thickened to the desired consistency.

Servings: Four to Eight

Preparation Time: Four minutes

Cooking Time: Low - six to eight hours

Casseroles

Crock-Pot® Dinner: Beef or Chicken

Ingredients

1 Whole/cut up chicken –or- legs and thighs OR a Beef Roast

2 Carrots

4 Potatoes

5 Ounces water

1 Can celery or cream of mushroom soup (10 ¾ ounce)

Directions

1) Cut the carrots into four-inch chunks. Put all of the ingredients

   into the Crock-Pot®.

2) Set the Pot and let it 'go.'

Servings: Four

Cooking Time: The high setting will cook the meal in six hours, or you can cook it all day using the low-temperature setting.

Squash 'N Chops

Ingredients

5 Pork (boneless) Port cutlets or chops

2 medium oranges

1 ¼ Pounds delicate/butternut squash

1/8 tsp. Ground red pepper

½ tsp. Garlic salt

¼ tsp. Each: Ginger, cloves, and cinnamon

Directions

1) Peel and slice the oranges. Peel and slice the squash lengthwise and discard the seeds. Cut the 'half' into sections ½-inches thick.

2) Flavor the pork with some garlic salt and red peppers. Use a 4- to 5- quart Crock-Pot® and place the chops/cutlets in the bottom.

3) Combine the ginger, cinnamon, and cloves in a small dish.

4) Top off the pork with the oranges along with the toppings in step 3.

5) Cover and cook.

Servings: 5

Cooking Time: Low for 4 hours

Lasagna Enchantment

This one has a few more steps, but it is so worth it—and it's easy.

Ingredients

2 Cans diced tomatoes (28-ounces) drained
Four finely chopped clove of garlic
2 Tbsp. oregano
½ tsp. salt
15-ounces fresh ricotta
¼ tsp. pepper
½ tsp. salt
½ C. shredded Parmesan cheese
1 (12-ounce) Package uncooked lasagna noodles
½ tsp. fresh (finely chopped) parsley – more if desired
2 C. spinach leaves (bagged is okay)
2 C. shredded Mozzarella cheese

Directions

1) Mix the garlic, drained tomatoes, pepper, salt, and oregano in a mixing container.

2) In another bowl, blend the parsley, Parmesan, and ricotta cheese.

3) Dip anywhere from 1/3 to ½ cup of the tomato combination on the base of the Crock-Pot®.

4) Layer the noodles, spinach, several dollops of the ricotta combo, and 1/3 to about ½ of the tomato combination. Sprinkle the mozzarella on the top of that section. Continue the process with the mozzarella on the top.

5) Close the lid on the Pot and let it do the work.

Servings: Six to Eight
Prep Time: 20 Minutes
Cook Time: High is 2 Hrs. or Low is 3 to 4 Hrs.

Sweet Potato Casserole

Ingredients
1 ½ C. applesauce
1 tsp. ground cinnamon
3 Tbsp. Margarine/butter
½ C. Toasted chopped nuts
2/3 C. Brown sugar
6 medium sweet potatoes

Directions

1) Peel and slice the potatoes cutting them into ½-inch bits and drop them into a 3 ½-quart Crock-Pot®.

2) In a separate dish, mix the brown sugar, cinnamon, melted butter, and applesauce. *Note:* Be sure you pack the brown sugar tight when it is measured.

3) Empty the mixture over the potatoes in the Pot.

4) When the potatoes are tender; you can top with the chopped nuts. Yummy!

Cooking Time: Six to Eight hours

Sides/Veggies

Slow Cooked Baked Potatoes

Ingredients

6 Baking Potatoes

Kosher Salt

Oil

Garnishes: Your choice

Directions

1) Prepare the potatoes with a good scrub and rinsing, but do not dry them.

2) Put each one in some foil while poking holes in each one using a fork.

3) Use a small amount of oil to drizzle over each one adding a sprinkle of salt, and close the foil.

4) To keep them from getting soggy, ball up several wads of foil into the cooker.

5) Layer the potatoes on the balls and cover. Leave them on warm in the Crock-Pot® until ready to serve.

Cooking Time: Low – Six to Eight Hours

Corn on the Cob

Ingredients

3 ears or 5 to 6 halves – Corn on the cob

Salt as needed

1/2 stick or ¼ cup of softened butter

Directions

1) Shuck and remove the silks from the corn; break them into halves.

2) Cover each one with butter and wrap individually in foil.

3) Wad some foil balls up in the base of the unit and add about 1-inch of water.

4) Put the potatoes into the Crock-Pot®, and cook for the allotted time.

Servings: 4

Preparation Time: Five minutes

Cooking Time: Use the high setting for two hours. *Note*: The cooking time may vary if you prepare the corn with another unit besides a 5 to 6-quart pot.

Ranch Mushrooms

Ingredients
½ Cup Melted butter
1 Pound fresh mushrooms
1 Package - ranch salad dressing mix
Instructions
1) Leave the mushrooms whole and wash them well.

2) Put them into the Crock-Pot®, adding the oil and ranch mix by drizzling it over the mushrooms.

3) Cover the Pot. It is best to stir once after hour one to blend the butter.

Servings: Six
Cooking Time: Low will have your mushrooms ready in three to four hours.

Sweet Potatoes

Ingredients

4 medium sweet potatoes

Optional Garnishes:

Brown Sugar, Butter, Mini Marshmallows

Directions

1) Clean and prepare the potatoes—thoroughly dry.

2) Use a fork and poke holes in each one, and double wrap them in aluminum foil.

3) Put them in the Crock-Pot®--cooking them the specified amount of time. If you are close to the kitchen; turn and flip the potatoes in the pot occasionally.

4) Once they are done, add the garnishes of your choice and serve.

Servings: Four
Preparation Time: Five Minutes
Cooking Time: The Low setting is used for 8 hrs. or the High setting for 4 hrs. (Times may vary depending on the size of the potatoes, but you will know when they are ready by how soft the potato is when you give it a squeeze.)

Chapter 5: Desserts – Snacks & Treats to Devour

Apple Dump Cake

Ingredients

Butter (1 Stick)

Yellow cake mix (1 box)

Apple pie filling (1 Can)

Directions

1) Empty the apple filling into the Crock-Pot®.

2) *Dump* in the mix and then the butter on top of the mix.

Cooking Time: Cook the cake in the Pot on the low setting for approximately four hours for best results.

Enjoy!

Applesauce

Ingredients

12 Apples

1 teaspoon juice (+) ¼ of the lemon peel

2 cinnamon sticks

Directions

1) Peel, core, and slice the apples. Put the apples, lemon peel, and sticks into the Crock-Pot®.

2) Provide a drizzle to the top with the juice and set the cooking timer.

3) When the treat is ready—throw the lemon peel and cinnamon sticks into the garbage.

4) Blend with a regular or immersion blender.

5) Chill for a few hours.

Cooking Time is five to seven hrs.

Peach Cobbler

Ingredients

1 White cake mix (not prepared)

6 Large peaches

1- Stick (½- Cup) softened butter

Directions

1) Peel and slice the peaches, and put them into the Crock-Pot®.

2) Blend the butter and cake mix using a pastry blender. You want a crumbly texture.

3) Sprinkle the mix over the peaches, and cook.

Enjoy with a bowl of ice cream.

Servings: Eight

Preparation Time: Fifteen minutes

Cooking Times on the high setting is two to three hours; whereas the Low cycle will extend for about four hours.

Cocktail Franks – Sweet and Sour

Ingredients

40- Ounces Pineapple chunks

2 Pounds cocktail franks

1 Cup each:

- Grape jelly

- Chili sauce

3 Tablespoons each:

- Prepared mustard

- Lemon juice

Directions

1) Mix the jelly, chili sauce, mustard, and lemon juice in the Pot, mixing it well.

2) Cover and use the high setting for fifteen to twenty minutes to blend the ingredients

3) Slice the franks into bite-sized pieces and add to the Crock-Pot®.

4) Pour in the drained chunks of pineapple.

Servings: 10

Cooking Times: High setting for two hours; *Low* setting for four hours.

Index for the Recipes

Chapter 2: Healthy Breakfast Recipes

- Boiled Eggs

- One-Hour Bread

- Breakfast Fiesta Delight

- Italian Sausage Scramble

The Sweeter Side of Breakfast

- Blueberry Steel Cut Oats

- Pumpkin Pie Oatmeal

- Pumpkin Butter

Chapter 3: Time-Saving Lunch Specialties

- Beef Tacos

- Root Beer & BBQ Chicken

- Stuffed Banana Peppers

- Crock-Pot® Taco Soup

Chapter 4: Dinner in a Hurry

Beef

- Meat for the Tacos

- Steak Pizzaiola

- Steak in the Pot

Chicken & Turkey

- Buffalo Chicken

- Caesar Chicken

- Cranberry Chicken

- French Onion Chicken

- Hawaiian Chicken

- Honey Mustard Chicken

- Chicken Italian Style

- Swedish Meatballs

- Sweet and Sour Chicken

- Creamy Taco Chicken

- Stuffed – Roasted Turkey

Fish

- Citrus Flavored Fish

- Salmon Bake

Pork

- BBQ Style Pork Steaks

- Pepsi® Roast

- Ranch Chops

- Ham in Cider Gravy

Casseroles

- Crock-Pot® Dinner: Beef or Chicken

- Squash 'N Chops

- Lasagna Enchantment

- Sweet Potato Casserole

Sides & Veggies
- Slow Cooked Baked Potatoes

- Corn on the Cob

- Ranch Mushrooms

- Sweet Potatoes

Chapter 5: Desserts to Devour

- Apple Dump Cake

- Applesauce

- Peach Cobbler

- Cocktail Franks – Sweet and Sour

CPSIA information can be obtained
at www.ICGtesting.com
Printed in the USA
LVHW041925081020
668360LV00004B/239